Our Journey Through Prostate Cancer

by

Jim Miller and Julia Miller

TABLE OF CONTENTS

APPRECIATION

That great oak tree's crash. But louder howls the storm. It wakes the young, urging them to live and grow. . . . Go forth life, into the light!

—Verte

This book is about our emotions, the pain of cancer and the joy of life, the release of energy and pent-up feelings. Only with the love and help of our family, our children, and our friends has this been made possible. We love you all so much. Thank you.

To Jim, my husband, you are a living miracle and the love of my life. Although I narrate our story, it is you who have lived with cancer and were willing to share our personal experience with others.

We are so grateful for our love and friendship. Our relationship is filled with energy from the healing and curing of Jim. We look forward to our future journeys together, to living together every day in body, mind, and soul.

A special appreciation goes to Dr. Peter Carroll, of the University of California at San Francisco (UCSF), for all his hours of dedicated care and his professional consult on the book. Additionally, the ongoing care of Dr. Mack Roach, also of UCSF; Margaret Arent; Michael Broffman; and Cindy Mack have given more to us than they will ever know.

PREFACE

When we are really honest with ourselves, we must admit our lives are all that really belong to us. So it is how we use our lives that determines the kind of men we are.

—Cesar Chavez

On a plane flight from San Francisco to Washington, D.C., an attractive man in his early thirties asked across the aisle, "What are you writing about?"

"Surviving cancer," I responded. "What kind?" he asked. Imagine the surprise on his face when I said prostate cancer.

It turned out that his father had had prostate cancer and, as a result, his prostate removed two years earlier. His father was still depressed, he said, because of complications with his urinary function and bladder control. "Since my father's illness, I have really started to think about what I can do to help prevent cancer and how to best treat it," said James, only 34 years old. "It's amazing how much more aware I am now that cancer has hit home."

It was a clear indication to me that writing this book was the right thing to do. James knew about the tough road that is prostate cancer, but most don't. More people need a guide with a personal perspective to help them navigate all the details, emotions, and options concerning prostate cancer. Hopefully, this story will help you gain some insight into the journey to healing and the experience of facing the disease and living victoriously through it.

For me, writing this book was cathartic. As I rehashed all the moments of my husband Jim's illness and transfered them to paper, they truly became things of the past, now living only in print and in our memories. They live to remind us of the value of life and love, and to teach others the path we took through this terrible disease to full healing and curing.

If you are reading this book, you most likely have prostate cancer or know someone who has prostate cancer, or you just may be concerned about the disease. This book will give you a personal account of the three-year healing process Jim and I lived through while he was undergoing treatment. It personalizes the experience and is intended to help you understand that if you are diagnosed with this initially frightening disease, you have some control over what will happen to you. It is intended to help you cope and make you or your loved one more likely to have a successful healing process.

We are not suggesting that, for a successful cure and healing, you follow the details of what we did, but at least this book will give you some options to consider. While it may be a difficult journey, the lessons you learn about life and love will be invaluable.

INTRODUCTION

The journey of a thousand miles must begin with one step.

—Lao-tzu

Below is a one-on-one interview with Jim about what it is like to discover you have prostate cancer and how it feels to live with the disease.

Q. What were you first thoughts when you found out you had cancer?

A. I guess my first thought was, "I could die," and it scared me so much I went into denial. I found myself saying, "It will be alright. No big deal. I can get through this." But inside I was fearful I would die.

Q. When was the first time you cried after learning you had cancer?

A. When I was driving to work the day after I found out it started to settle in, "This was not a mistake." I did not know what it meant, but I knew that a PSA of 39.5 was serious, so I was scared and didn't know what was going to happen to me—if I would die. Tears just came from nowhere. The emotions later in the week were even more intense. It's the crying I remember the most. I was crying about dying and knowing I didn't want to suffer a long time if I was going to die. It was just so sad—I couldn't keep myself from crying. I was too young to die, and I had too many things I still wanted to do.

Q. What was the worst part of the treatments?

A. The uncertainty of knowing whether they were going to work. The fear is worse than the treatments, even though they aren't anything to be delighted about either.

Q. How did prostate cancer impact your sexuality?

A. The treatments reduced my libido, to the point of having no desire for sex. However, the drugs on the market today helped my sexual performance, and, fortunately, I did not have a problem with total impotence. It is hard to accept.

Q. What worries you most, now that you are finished with your treatment?

A. My biggest fear is that my PSA will begin to rise and the cancer will return—especially to another part of my body. That fear never goes away.

Q. Is it ever over?

A. No, no, it is an ongoing war in which I do everything I can to fight back, including ongoing medical care, nutrition, exercise, and more.

Q. What would you tell every man about prostate cancer?

A. Get a PSA at age forty, unless there is a history of the disease in your family—and then get it earlier. I know the medical community says fifty, but I was in my late forties when I found out and wish I had known earlier."

Q. What would you tell every caregiver about prostate cancer?

A. Love him [the person with prostate cancer], and be supportive of whatever has to be done to heal and cure.

Q. What will you do if your prostate cancer returns?

A. Work with my doctors to determine our strategy for the next phase of healing and curing. There are always options.

Q. What good has come from having prostate cancer?

A. It has given me the opportunity to reevaluate my life and what is most important: living life well. I find I've changed from doing things I always felt I "should be doing" to living my life how I want to live it.

One beautiful day, Jim was driving his sporty white convertible on his way to taking care of his daily business. He checked his voice mail and found the usual calls from the boss, the staff, outside suppliers, and the like. However, one call was unusual. Jim had recently had a routine annual physical, and his doctor called with the results, leaving a rather cryptic message: "Jim, please call me. We need to discuss the results of one of your tests." The next day, we found out that Jim had prostate cancer. Even though he had no symptoms and was under fifty years old, somehow he had this dreadful disease. Not only did he have prostate cancer, but his cancer was inoperable because it had spread in his body beyond his prostate.

The news was overwhelming, numbing, and frightening all at once. Everything seemed to happen so fast now we had to consciously slow down to let the gamut of our emotions flow. We had no idea what was to become of our lives, but we were certain of one thing: We wanted Jim to be one hundred percent healed and cured. We didn't know how we would accomplish this, but we believed it was possible. And we were going to do whatever it would take to make this happen, no matter what.

Jim and I rolled up our sleeves and went to battle with this inoperable prostate cancer. We were committing body, mind, and soul to healing and curing Jim.

Healing and Curing

One important lesson that we learned early on was the difference between healing and curing. We had never thought of it before, but there is a significant difference between being healed and being cured. Citing Webster's dictionary, there is a distinction:

> **Cure** is defined as "to deal with in a way that eliminates or rectifies."
> **Heal** is defined as "to make whole and to restore health."

We decided that we wanted both for Jim, but most importantly we wanted Jim to be healed. This meant that in addition to our external resources, we would have to go deep within ourselves and mine all of our internal resources. Jim would have to deal with all aspects of himself—husband, father, business executive, male, and human being. He would have to repair the damage that was done over the years and work to regain his health and create a reality where he could be a totally healthy man and remain cancer-free.

But, in fact, we need both healing and curing efforts when we are seriously ill with a life-threatening disease. Thus, we considered taking advantage of healing practices from a variety of sources, rather than putting all our eggs in the traditional Western medicine basket. Merely counting on the procedures and drugs that were being suggested by our Western doctors did not intuitively seem to be enough to tackle the challenge we had before us.

We explored alternative options with our friends and doctors. We combed bookstores, attended seminars, and searched the Internet to learn what else was out there that could help Jim.

We talked about it, cried about it, worried about it, and finally decided we would be open to almost anything and everything to create a healing and nurturing environment for Jim. While neither of us had ever participated in Eastern medicine or alternative-healing options, we went after them with all our energy and resources. Jim pursued a complete regimen of acupuncture, herbs and vitamins, exercise, fasting, mental support, visualization, and more.

Committing to Change

Our healing journey took us from Honolulu to San Francisco to Ann Arbor (for a brief symposium) and back to San Francisco. It caused us to change our work habits; incorporate a new, intensive healing regimen into our lives; modify our diets; exercise more; rest more; and learn about all sorts of things we never thought would enter our lives. Right away, I decided to work alongside Jim to support all the changes he would need to make. We developed an extensive healing action plan for Jim with the input of doctors, professionals, trainers, and ourselves. Based on outside input and our own lifestyle, we took their recommendations and modified them to suit our individual needs. We knew we had to believe our plan was the best it could be. We also knew we needed to commit ourselves to the plan with all the energy and resources we had at our disposal.

Jim's cancer forced him to do some serious soul-searching. He asked himself the tough questions about life: what he wanted from it, what he would do to keep it, and what kind of person he wanted to be in the universe. While his life seemed too precarious at times, the desire and will to survive grew stronger, and his love of himself and others grew deeper and richer. By getting more in touch with who he was, he was able to let others experience his love and leadership firsthand. Jim did this by committing himself to changing many aspects of who he was prior to learning he had cancer. He thought deeply about what might have made him ill. He questioned what made him tick and realized he had always kept too much inside. Such repression of his feelings would no longer be acceptable anymore. He was going to have to address his past, but, even more importantly, focus on the here and now. He was now going to do whatever was in his power to accept his thoughts and to express his feelings, including those of disappointment, anger, and jealousy. This would enable him to spend time thinking about healing and releasing many of those other emotions into the world—out of his body. Jim also had to learn to reach out and build a network of support for himself from other cancer patients, doctors, healing practitioners, and friends and family.

Committing his body to the healing process meant that Jim could no longer afford to sleep three or four hours a night because of a hectic work schedule. Sleeping and resting would become an important part of the day: His body needed time to recover from the drugs and treatments, which zapped his energy. The way he treated his body was to be a critical force in fighting the cancer, and he focused on multiple ways to support his body in its efforts to heal.

I found it necessary to make changes—eating and cooking healthfully to set the stage for Jim, and keeping up with his sleeping schedule for support and my own rest. Fighting cancer is emotionally draining for partners. Periods of exhaustion overcame me, and I was more susceptible to illness at this time. Workouts, lots of sleep, and eating well are vital for both patient and partner.

Emerging Victorious

Cancer is a personal struggle for all involved. Jim and I believe it is part of the wider struggle for life, for acceptance, for forgiveness, for our bodies, for our minds—a struggle for our souls. That Jim's life was at risk was devastating to both of us, but we were able to work through the pain together, emerging stronger and with more belief than ever in the power of the human spirit. As his wife, partner, lover, and head cheerleader, I learned that I had a vital role in the outcome.

Jim's struggle with cancer is like a marathon of a life experience, and we are making it through, still breathing and still very much alive. Jim has his PSA monitored every three months. It remains below .18. We have time to go until we get the official all-clear sign from the doctors. But we know in our hearts that after more than one thousand days of treatment, Jim is healed and cured.

We have emerged from the journey more in love and in appreciation of life than ever before. We wish the same for you.

THE CIRCLE OF HEALING

We are like the shining sun, and our sickness, like passing clouds which appear to extinguish the sun's ray. The wise person who gazes at the dull gray sky knows that, in reality, the sun still shines brightly behind the veil of the clouds. All that is needed to uncover its radiance is a clear, strong wind.

—Buddhist teaching

Our journey through prostate cancer led us through a process that allowed us to cope with all that was happening to us. The best way to describe this process is as a circle, what I affectionately refer to as the Circle of Healing.

The Circle of Healing includes all the steps we took to enable us to actively manage and participate in the entire healing journey. It starts with detection of the illness and then moves to determining appropriate treatment options. Then comes the active involvement of committing physical and emotional resources to the healing process. The final phase is one that never ends; it includes following up to ensure the individualized healing plan is still working.

One of the results of Jim's having had cancer is that we learned to separate the noise of what seemed urgent from what was truly important to us. Because we were facing the possibility of Jim's dying from the disease, we became deeply self-reflective, especially Jim. He was always the type of person who had difficulty saying no to anything or anyone, but he realized he was going to have to start to do this. He was the type of person who was always overextended because of being torn in so many directions. What he realized was that he was going to have to say no to some of the demands made on him so that he could use the weakened energy he had to heal and cure himself. He needed to reconsider his approach to life and break some old habits and learn new ones. He realized that to come through this disease totally healed and cured he was going to have to give up things that were not positive for his well-being or that demanded more of him then he could give. He became very cautious of overcommitting to family, friends, and work so he could, for the first time in his life, put himself first.

The following diagram illustrates how we approached Jim's prostate cancer, but be aware that the Circle of Healing we created for Jim was particular to his struggle and that it may be different for every person. Nothing is prescribed. The Circle of Healing below shows a way through the fear and uncertainty, coming from the challenge of dealing with cancer. We knew we needed to approach this challenge in a way that we could believe in with our hearts. The Circle of Healing became a clear pathway for us to understand where this journey was taking us, and how we would be able to live with it and through it.

The interaction of the Circle of Healing is the harmony of recognizing the interconnection of body, mind, and soul for healing. The circle is comparable to a ring, which has neither a beginning nor an end. Each person with cancer can find themselves somewhere in the Circle of Healing. It is simply a means by which any-

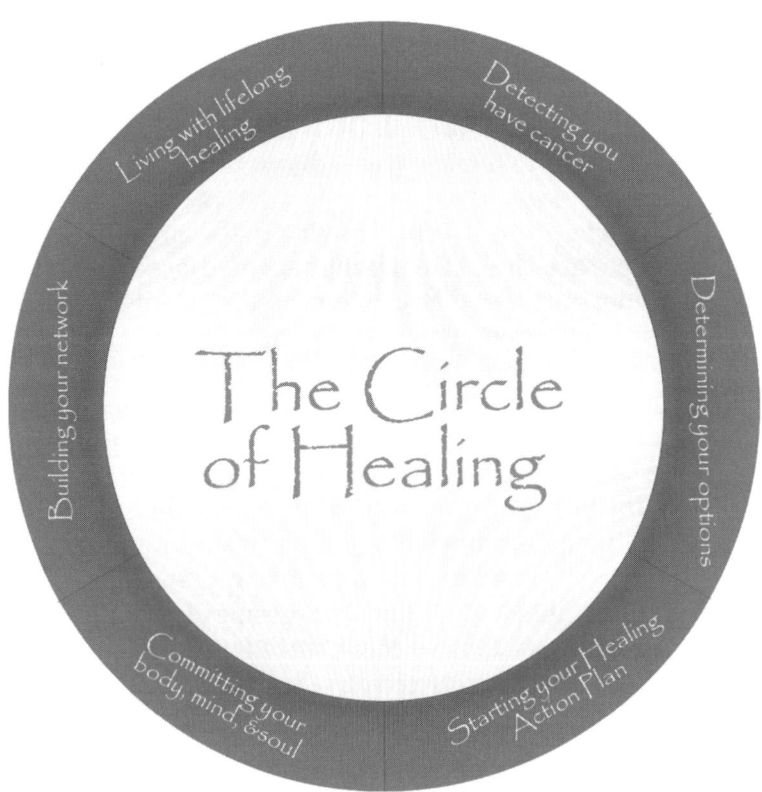

one can understand the process of living through a disease such as cancer and its treatment. Through creating a circle of this kind, we can start to accept the ongoing nature of healing and the need to continue living our lives.

This is not "the five steps to curing" but a journey of healing to be taken as you trek through prostate cancer. The journey starts when people become aware that they or one of their loved ones has the disease. The next step in the journey occurs as one determines healing options, and is followed by the development and execution of a healing plan. This can be as simple as a mental roadmap or as detailed as a step-by-step outline of one's treatment plan. The important point here was for us to establish a clear vision of what we wanted out of our healing process. Lastly, the process evolves to the completion of the circle. At this stage, we realized the need to commit to lifelong healing, having found the desire to commit to total well-being is critical.

We learned that an individualized plan was required, because no one knew as much about us as we did. Jim and others who have been successful have taken an active part in the healing process by committing themselves to the plan they created just for themselves. This is your life, your reality, and we believe it is possible to actively help to manifest the outcome you desire. While cancer and its impact are so disorienting, to overcome the disease requires, ironically, that you remain rational and logical in order to make the best possible decisions for treatment. This is not easy, as your mind is racing, contemplating all the options, and, at the same time, fearing the results. It is like nothing we have ever experienced or, hopefully, will ever experience again.

The Circle of Healing requires full engagement. The commitment manifests itself in a healing action plan for body, mind, and soul. By doing this, a healthy environment for the body is created to heal, and the mind can communicate to body and soul. There is a complete internal dialogue about total healing and curing. Lastly, the soul of the person needs to be willing to accept and guide the body and mind along a path that will enable complete healing to occur. By committing to a personalized healing action plan with your entire body, mind, and soul, you may find you will have to modify your lifestyle. You can empower yourself to do this, to create the best healthful living environment in which to heal and cure. While in the experience, you may begin to realize that we have to heal ourselves from within, from the inside out. The goal is to create an environment in our body, where we can spontaneously heal with the assistance of all the external forces. These external forces include the potential sources of learning and treatment from modern, ancient, and alternative medicine and methods.

While engaging in the healing process, one fact becomes evident: No one makes this journey alone, nor should you expect to do so. Developing a powerful network of family, friends, doctors, and other cancer survivors will provide the foundation on which to build a proactive healing action plan. The network can be as big or as small as is right for each individual. One important part of the network is other patients with prostate cancer. Within this, there is an opportunity to share the experience with others who truly are experiencing firsthand the same or similar experiences. Additionally, their perspective can help to frame their view of their journey with personal anecdotes and challenges. Support groups have been shown to improve long-term survival rates of patients by over thirty percent.

When you learn that you or someone you love has prostate cancer, the first few weeks are especially difficult because intense emotion is mixed with the physical uncertainty of the progress of the disease. With prostate cancer, the process is even more profound because the disease impacts a man's sexuality and, therefore, the very essence of his masculinity and who he is—just as breast cancer does for women. The first step in the Circle of Healing is detecting and diagnosing prostate cancer. While this might seem self-evident, there are millions of men around the world today who have prostate cancer and are not aware of it. There are a variety of tests you can take to detect prostate cancer.

The next step in the Circle of Healing is determining what healing and treatment options to consider. This sounds like a relatively simple step, but it is one of the most critical parts of engaging in the entire process of healing. The combination of treatments and healing options available to you are varied and can range from watchful waiting (measuring your cancer levels over time with no active treatment), to surgery, or even to participation in a clinical trial. We learned that being prepared to spend energy to determine a proactive treatment plan that was right for us was critical and would save Jim's life.

Developing and implementing a healing plan tailored just for you comes next. This book covers all areas you might want to consider—diet, exercise, alternative treatment options, and stress management. In creating your plan, you must examine all areas of your life and identify where healthful changes can be made.

The remaining step in the Circle of Healing process is critical because it requires continued action and lifelong follow-up. Anyone who has had cancer must monitor his health to ensure successful management of the disease and to prevent reoccurrence in the future.

This entire healing process is an ongoing course of action that we go through to emerge from cancer as more complete and total humans than before. No matter what the final outcome, this journey and process can lead to a better and fuller life with or without cancer.

PART ONE

PROSTATE CANCER ENTERS OUR LIVES

DETECTION AND DIAGNOSIS

Look and you will find. What is unsought will go undetected.

—Sophocles

Life Before Cancer

For over twenty years, Jim was busy keeping up with the demands of being a senior executive and raising a family. He was so driven to become the ultimate caretaker of others that he forgot to take care of himself. Working for the Duty Free Stores division of LVMH (Louis Vuitton Moet Henessey) in Honolulu, Jim had people from around the world contacting him at all hours of the day. Each day he would get up between 3:00 A.M. and 4:00 A.M. to answer e-mail from the night before for an hour or two. Then he'd go for a quick run, shower, gulp down a glass of orange juice, gobble a bagel, and dash out the door. He was usually in the office by 7:00 A.M. and did not get home until around 7:00 P.M. In the evening, he'd eat a quick dinner, read the paper, and be asleep by 10:00. On nights before an event or when a major initiative was due, he could be up until midnight and sleep just three hours. In addition, his job required him to spend twenty to thirty percent of his time traveling, which included some overseas trips to places like London, Florence, Paris, or Singapore—beautiful places, but stressful trips.

Ultimately Jim's body became overwhelmed and "dis-eased" with such an extreme schedule. Initially, he had no symptoms of prostate cancer, with the exception of infrequent back stiffness and fatigue. However, as most of us do, he explained it away with comments like, "I worked late, and I'm tired," or, "I was in a meeting most of the day, which is why I'm stiff." We should have listened to Jim's body earlier. It was calling out to us, screaming, "I'm exhausted and overworked. Please let me rest!" Jim was driving his body and his mind much too hard for too long, and not reenergizing himself.

The Day That Changed Our Lives

One day, after a routine exam, our family doctor called and asked Jim to come in to review some test results. Fearing the results, Jim wasted no time and set up an appointment for the next day. That evening, the appointment was only a casual part of our usual dinner conversation. Jim mentioned, with slight apprehension, that there might be a problem, so we agreed that I should go along to hear firsthand what this was about. Little did we know what was in store for us. That day changed the course of our lives—a disorienting dilemma, as Jim likes to say.

While we were driving to Dr. Chun's office, I struggled with a sense of fear that kept creeping into my thoughts. What was this all about? Oh, it will be fine—my usual optimistic self-talk kicked in to calm my nerves. Jim looks so healthy. If there is something wrong, it will only be a minor problem. By the time we walked into the office, both of our hearts were racing. The nervousness went beyond the issue of the test results. We sensed there was much more during this meeting. It was the impact of the results, how we lived our lives, and the fear of what might change beyond our control that made us so tense.

The assistant called us in and we both sat there listening to Dr. Chun explain Jim's test results. Jim had a PSA of over 39. Any level over 4 is a potential problem, especially at his age. Without any knowledge of the degree of his illness, we knew that this was serious, very serious. Still, Dr. Chun was careful to say that he was only a general practitioner and that Jim needed to take another test to confirm the initial results. Dr. Chun was an excellent general practitioner, as it turns out.

Maybe the test results are wrong, I thought anxiously. You know the "false positive" stories you hear about: Someone is told he's sick, but the test results turn out to be incorrect. I was in serious denial, and Jim was in serious disbelief—there is a difference. I was afraid of cancer, and Jim couldn't believe that he, Jim Miller, really had cancer. There was an awkward moment, none of us knowing what to say. They don't teach you how to deal with this kind of real-life experience in school. Dr. Chun and I waited for Jim to speak first. Typical of Jim, his cool, calm executive side took over.

"Dr. Chun, how serious is this?" said Jim, shocked.
"Jim, this is serious," he replied, looking us both dead on.

"Am I going to die from this?" Jim said, beckoning with his hands, his mouth agape.

"There are so many factors involved, and we will need to run more tests to understand how fast the cancer is growing." Dr. Chun stood up and placed his hands in his pocket.

"What do we do next?" Jim said, shaking his head back and forth, searching inwardly.

"I'll set up some more diagnostic tests. I also recommend you go see Dr. Chinn. He's one of our best urologists." Dr. Chun was as serious as he had the capacity to be. This was real.

"Okay," Jim replied softly, concerned.

So that was it. No actual answers, no treatment, no clear next step. I was so frustrated, hot, and a little dizzy. My mind was reeling. Jim's mind was reeling. Didn't the doctors know what to do? Don't we pay them to tell us what we should do in these situations? Aren't they the experts? We hardly expected to find out about such a serious situation in this small, unpretentious doctor's office.

It was almost surreal, like it wasn't happening to us. Jim was numb. I felt like I was sitting above the office and looking down on the situation, suddenly removed from it. Most likely, this response was self-protection, a coping mechanism.

We left the doctor's office quietly. I remember walking over to the car in the parking lot and thinking, This isn't happening. Look at Jim—he's the picture of health. He runs every day, he isn't overweight, and he feels great.

I looked at our surroundings: gorgeous Honolulu, one of the most beautiful places in the world. All of a sudden, the health of Jim's body and our minds was fading from being as healthy as the lush island that we called home.

As we got in the car, I started to cry. When I looked at Jim I thought of those cells inside of him, those bad, potentially deadly cancer cells. How many were they? Let's just cut the cancer out; let's get rid of this.

That night, we cried together in bed. Without understanding everything, we knew this was bad. We were both scared, scared of what we now knew and even more afraid of what the future might have in store.

The next morning, I was on the phone to make an appointment with a specialist who could give us much more specific answers to the hundreds of questions running through our minds.

Being productive at this time was exceedingly helpful in processing this new situation. It was awful, but preoccupying your mind was a great benefit; it made you feel like you were doing something good, and that was important.

Jim was one of the lucky ones. His primary-care physician paid attention, questioned him about his family history, and decided proactively to test him early, before he was fifty. Not everyone is so lucky. It's crucial that men make their overall health—and the health of their prostate—their own responsibility. Prostate cancer can strike before you are fifty, and early detection is vital to a positive long-term prognosis of prostate and overall health.

Screening Is Critical

Dr. Chun believed that Jim most likely developed prostate cancer over many years. This was extremely upsetting and frustrating for us. In spite of all the advances in modern medicine, how could this happen? This aggravated us for a long time, and we kept asking ourselves why we didn't learn about this earlier. Jim had an annual physical with personal referrals and highly trained doctors, but that was not enough. Sometimes this type of cancer just happens despite everyone's desire to prevent it. Jim and I didn't let the frustration stop us from moving forward. It was too late now for us to wish for early detection, we just had to deal with the situation as it was.

In most cases, prostate cancer is a relatively slow-growing form of the disease. Because it normally affects men in their later years, patients can often live with the disease without any impact on their life expectancy. Thus, there are some doctors who believe screening and testing are not necessary. Based on our personal experience, we cannot disagree more emphatically with this approach. Detection based solely on symptoms can be difficult, because the disease can grow without any symptoms or effect on bodily functions such as urination and sexual function.

From our perspective, all men middle-aged and older (fifty plus) must be sure to get tested regularly. This is most commonly done with a simple prostate-specific antigen (PSA) blood test. PSA is a protein produced by the prostate gland and found in low levels in the blood. Its level rises in some men who have prostate cancer, benign prostatic hyperplasia, or prostatitis. The higher the level, the greater the potential problem. In a healthy man, the PSA level is under four, and ideally below two. A level of twenty or over indicates a serious problem. A PSA blood test should be administered regularly after the age of fifty. In cases where there is a family history of prostate cancer, a man should be tested even earlier. Early diagnosis can improve survival rates dramatically—as much as fifty percent.

Continuous symptoms such as lower back pain and painful or burning urination need to be recognized as potential early warning signs of a problem. Early signs of prostate cancer may include:

- Difficulty starting urination
- Difficulty holding back urination
- Inability to urinate
- A need to urinate frequently
- Painful ejaculation
- Blood in urine or semen
- Pain or stiffness in the lower back, hips, or upper thighs

If your father or other relatives had prostate cancer, be sure to get tested regularly. Your chances of getting prostate cancer are fifty percent greater. Be sure to get screened with a PSA test before the age of fifty, based on input from your doctor. It just might save your life. At least you will sleep more soundly, without worrying there may be something seriously wrong.

Ten Things to Do When the Doctor Says It's Cancer

No trumpets sound when the important decisions of our life are made. Destiny is made known silently.

—Agnes de Mille

Perhaps you or your loved one has just heard the same gut-wrenching news that Jim and I heard. You may feel a whole range of emotions, from denial to anger to profound fear. Your feelings are a natural part of the process, and they are crucial to helping you deal with the difficult situation. But whatever you do at this painful juncture, do not believe that you are helpless. There are some positive steps you can take, both mentally and practically, that can help you take the next step forward.

1. **Believe the diagnosis.** It's natural to go through a period of denial. However, the bottom line is that, unfortunately, you most likely have cancer. Begin to accept it and start the healing process. Jim did not believe that he had cancer after just one test; we hoped it was a mistake. But when the second set of more extensive tests came back, there was no denying it was cancer—sad, but true.

2. **Get a second opinion.** Choosing a treatment plan is a huge decision to make, and you should review as many options as possible before doing so. It is not insulting to your doctor to ask for a second opinion, and it will help you make the most informed decision. The best way to get a second opinion is by asking your doctor for the name of another professional. You can also call your insurance company or your local hospital for a referral.

3. **Take charge of your healing plan.** No one cares more about your healing than you and your family. No one will develop a complete treatment plan for you. You need to do it yourself. By engaging in this, you are doing a very important thing for yourself. You are empowering yourself to take charge of your body and your health. Congratulations.

4. **Reach out to people just like you.** Talk to someone who has had prostate cancer, and learn from his experiences. If you are a family member of someone with prostate cancer, seek out others who have also supported their loved one through this. Share the pain, and realize that there are others who can help. There are many ways to do this. Your local hospital may have a cancer resource center, or you can go online to contact organizations like USTOO! or PAACT (see Appendix, Valuable Resources).

5. **Commit yourself to healing.** The process starts when you commit yourself wholeheartedly—your thoughts, words, and actions—to healing. This can only happen when you allow yourself to accept what is happening to you and stop fighting the reality of your situation. Your commitment must also extend to your lifestyle—make

healing your life's focus, and direct a significant amount of your energy toward supporting your healing process through positive change in your life.

6. **Prepare for a marathon, not a sprint.** The healing process will not be over in a day, a week, a month, or even a year. You have entered a lifelong event, and you must pace yourself emotionally and physically. You'll need to get plenty of rest for your body to combat the cancer, and other lifestyle changes you make during treatment will most likely need to continue for the rest of your life.

7. **Have a "big life" day.** After reviewing a treatment plan with your doctor, take a day to fully think through your chosen healing process. Write it down, discuss it with family, make your decision based on what is right for you, and commit yourself completely to active healing. This day should be a quiet day, when you have few distractions and your loved ones are close by for support if you need them.

8. **Learn as much as you can.** By learning about what will potentially happen to you, you can cope more effectively and manage your fear. There are many places to access free information, such as the Internet, or you can purchase relevant books and magazines. The appendix of this book lists over 100 resources, books, and Web sites as potential places to start.

9. **Stop doing the things you dislike.** At times like this, it is important to take stock of what may be fueling your illness, causing the "dis-ease" in your life. Replace the things that you dislike or that cause a significant amount of stress with those that you love to do and that make you feel good. *"Saying no can be the ultimate self-care" — Claudia Black.*

10. **See yourself as a healthy, healed person.** We believe that ultimately the individual heals and cures his own body with the help of others. Doctors enable this to happen by contributing drugs, surgery, and other therapies to your cancer-fighting arsenal. You need to first believe that healing is possible for you in order to make it happen. Try to picture yourself fully healed, healthy, and happy. How are you different than you are today? Do you look different, act different, sound different? Do you think

differently? What will it take for you to see yourself as healthy and healed?

There are many other things you will do on your healing journey, but this list is a good start to help you mentally prepare for this ultimate life challenge.

Testing and Diagnosis

Jim initially had a PSA blood test as a part of his annual physical. It was then that we learned he had a PSA of 39. Afterwards, he had a multitude of tests performed, including a PSA and a DRE (digital rectal exam), by each doctor he visited. Because of the seriousness of his illness, he had an extensive biopsy done to determine how aggressive the tumor was in and around the prostate. Additionally, he had a ProstaScint scan, a TRUS (trans rectal ultrasound), and an MRI (magnetic resonance imaging) as the doctors tried to determine the best potential treatment for him.

Prostate cancer is diagnosed primarily through a combination of two widely used diagnostic tests—PSA and DRE. The initial PSA blood test is crucial to understanding how serious the cancer may be. The DRE is a procedure in which a doctor feels for a tumor or any unusual nodules on the prostate by inserting a gloved finger into the rectum.

A PSA of 4 ng/ml or below is less suggestive of prostate cancer. The actual cutoff value is somewhat dependent on your age. A higher PSA level by itself does not necessarily mean that you have prostate cancer, and a lower PSA level does not necessarily mean that you do not have prostate cancer. Be sure to ask your doctor to explain how the results from other tests can provide you with a clearer insight into your specific potential for prostate cancer.

A DRE enables your doctor to feel the size, shape, and texture of your prostate and nearby organs to determine if you may have a prostate or rectal disorder. However, you can have prostate cancer without having a palpable tumor (a tumor the doctor can feel), and, conversely, palpable nodules or abnormalities are not always prostate cancer. Again, this gets complicated; so make sure you understand this information.

Depending on the initial PSA test or your symptoms, your doctor will probably recommend one or more additional tests to understand the magnitude and potential growth rate of your cancer, and to help predict the success of various treatment options.

If your doctor finds a palpable tumor during DRE, he or she may advise you to have a biopsy of your prostate in an attempt to make a more accurate diagnosis. Your doctor may use TRUS to guide the biopsy needles and/or to help establish the volume of the prostate to determine the PSAD (PSA density). PSAD measures the correlation between the PSA level and the size and weight of the prostate as estimated by an ultrasound examination. With cancer, the PSA level may increase out of proportion to the size of the prostate, and the PSAD level will therefore increase.

It is important to know that none of these tests or procedures can deliver results that are 100 percent accurate. However, a combination of several tests can give doctors adequate understanding of the nature of the cancer for diagnostic purposes.

Jim's experience of going through these various diagnostic tests involved minor to moderate discomfort. Prior to taking the ProstaScint scan, Jim had to drink a gallon of green, slightly radioactive liquid. The radioactive particles attach themselves to potential cancer hot spots so the doctor can determine if the cancer has metastasized. Drinking the liquid was not easy to do, because the stuff doesn't taste good, and it's an enormous amount to drink the evening before the test. Unfortunately, in Jim's case hot spots were found in the lymph nodes in his pelvic region.

During the MRI, Jim was able to sleep with "long blinks," the time when his eyelids were so heavy they just had to close as if he were awake and asleep at the same time. Therefore, the experience for him was a fact-finding event, not an uncomfortable, confining one, as it is for many people, especially if they have claustrophobic tendencies. He was offered a sedative, but he didn't feel he needed it. Taking a sedative during this experience can be very helpful for patients who have claustrophobia or dislike being confined. Additionally, at certain medical facilities, there are now new MRI machines that are not as ominous and engulfing, so check with your doctor.

Another important test for the initial diagnosis was an examination of the prostate tissue. This exam is done via a biopsy. The biopsy from the TRUS process is painful, because the doctor has to insert a needle into the prostate and surrounding area to gather small tissue samples. Those samples are then examined by a pathologist to determine how aggressive and well-differentiated the cancer cells are. This is an important part of learning about the overall grade of the cancer. Jim's had a Gleason score of 8, with cancer on both sides of his prostate, making the grade four plus four (4 + 4). As far as the volume of the cancer cells, his right side had more cancer than his left side. Additionally, the cancer had spread throughout his seminal vesicles and in lymph nodes. This became important later on, as we explored treatment options.

The following chart defines each test and describes what the doctor intends to learn from the results. You should be sure to get the most complete testing initially, so the best possible treatment plan can be developed. Each man has a prostate cancer that is unique to him, based on his body and the particular type of prostate cancer cells.

A GUIDE TO COMMON TESTS

	Tests/ Examinations	**The Test Details**
Physical Tests and Exams	Digital Rectal Examination (DRE)	Insertion of a gloved lubricated finger into the rectum to feel the prostate.
	Chest X-ray	An image of the lungs that can show whether cancer has spread to the lung cavity.
	ProstaScint Scan	By injecting a radioisotope (a radioactive material) into the blood stream, which attaches itself to the cancer, and by using a gamma-ray camera, the location of prostate cancer, if any, in your body can be determined.

Tests/ Examinations	The Test Details
Bone scan	A picture that can show whether cancer has spread to bone.
Transrectal ultrasonography (TRUS)	A picture of the prostate and nearby body parts that is produced by soundwaves from an instrument inserted into the rectum.
Computed tomography (CT)	A picture produced by computer X-rays that shows the prostate and other nearby parts of the body
Intravenous pyelogram (IVP)	An X-ray of the kidneys, ureters, and bladder that is taken after the patient has been injected with a special dye.
Magnetic resonance imaging (MRI)	A picture produced by a computer and a high-powered magnet that shows the prostate and other nearby areas of the body.
RT-PCR	Can determine the presence of very small numbers of prostate cancer cells.
Serum acid phosphate test	Helps determine whether or not the prostate cancer has spread beyond the prostate and seminal vesicle capsule (normal range: 0.5–1.9 U/L)

	Tests/ Examinations	The Test Details
	Alkaline phosphatase test	Can determine whether the prostate cancer has spread to the bone (normal range: 90–239 U/L).
Blood Tests	Prostate-specific antigen (PSA)	A protein in blood that often increases in cases of prostate cancer and other prostate diseases. This test is useful both in diagnosis and follow-up of prostate cancer.
Tissue Samples	Prostate biopsy (determines Gleason grade)	The removal and examination under a microscope of a small sample of a prostate tumor to determine whether it contains cancer cells.
	Pelvic node dissection (also called lymphadenectomy)	A procedure used to determine whether prostate cancer has spread. This test is typically done during surgery to remove the prostate.

Please reference the glossary in the back of the book for a more detailed explanation of any term.

Ask your doctors to provide you with as much information as you need to feel comfortable with these tests and their results. After all, these people are being paid by you and your insurance company to help you through this experience. If you do not reach out to them, they may not be thoughtful enough to inform you of all the details of your disease. With complete information and understanding of your condition, you can help your doctors design the proper treatment plan.

Determining the Grade and Stage

If the diagnosis of prostate cancer is confirmed, your cancer will be assigned a grade and stage to identify the degree of your illness. The grade indicates the aggressiveness and growth rate of the cancer cells. The stage indicates the magnitude of cancer: how large the tumor is, whether it is contained within the prostate and, if not, how far it has spread. These are important variables to determine the type of treatment plan you need.

Most doctors use the Gleason grading system, which is based on the microscopic appearance of cells extracted from the prostate during biopsy. Your Gleason grade is determined by the shape and arrangement—the "architecture"—of your cells. The least aggressive cancer cells closely resemble normal cells. They are well differentiated, meaning they look clearly defined as individual cells under a microscope. The most aggressive cancer cells lump together in a shapeless mass and are poorly differentiated.

The Gleason scale includes three additional grade levels between these two extremes, for a total of five grades. To assign a grade to your tumor, the pathologist identifies the two most common patterns of cells in your biopsy (the primary and secondary patterns) and assigns a grade to each. These two grade levels are then added to determine your total Gleason score. The lowest total Gleason score is two (1 + 1), and the highest equals 10 (5 + 5). Scores of 4 or less indicate low-grade prostate cancers, which tend to be slower growing, and scores of 7 to 10 indicate high-grade cancers, which are often highly aggressive and faster growing. However, the Gleason score must be considered within the context of other data, including the tumor's stage and your PSA level.

Initial staging (determining the stage of your cancer prior to starting any treatment) usually combines results from the DRE (digital rectal exam), your PSA level, and the estimated tumor volume, based on the results of the TRUS. Additionally, your Gleason score and other tests may indicate whether or not your cancer has spread.

To help you better understand the fancy terms, *staging* is an important variable, just like the grade of the cancer. Staging is usually defined by the current international staging system for prostate cancer, called the TNM (tumornodemetastasis) system.

The *T* refers to the extent of the original tumor in the prostate, the *N* to the lymph nodes in the pelvic region, and the *M* to the presence or absence of distant metastases (whether the cancer has spread beyond the prostate to other parts of the body). The detailed chart below was provided by the National Institute for Health and describes the complete TNM staging system.

STAGING		
	Primary Tumor (T)	**Primary Tumor, Pathologic (pT)**
TX	Primary tumor cannot be assessed	pT2	Organ confined
TO	No evidence of primary tumor	pT2a	Unilateral
		pT2b	Bilateral
T1	Clinically an apparent tumor not palpable or visible by imaging		
T1a	Tumor incidental histologic finding in 5% or less of tissue resected	pT3	Extraprostatic extension
T1b	Tumor incidental histologic finding in more than 5% of tissue resected	pT3a	Extraprostatic extension
		pT3b	Seminal vesicle invasion
T1c	Tumor identified by needle biopsy (e.g., because of elevated PSA)		
T2	Palpable tumor confined within prostate		
T2a	Tumor involves one lobe	pT4	Invasion of bladder, rectum
T2b	Tumor involves both lobes		
T3	Tumor extends through the prostatic capsule		
T3a	Extracapsular extension (unilateral or bilateral) assessed		
T3b	Tumor invades seminal vesicle(s)		

Primary Tumor (T)		Regional Lymph Nodes (N)	
T4	Tumor is fixed or invades adjacent structures other than seminal vesicles: bladder neck, external sphincter, rectum	NX	Regional lymph nodes cannot be assessed
		N0	No regional lymph node metastasis
		N1	Metastasis in regional lymph node and nodes
		Distant Metastasis (M)	
		MX	Distant metastasis cannot be assessed
		M0	No distant metastasis
		M1	Distant metastasis
		M1a	Nonregional lymph nodes
		M1b	Bone(s)
		M1c	Other site(s)

The following chart shows risk levels for the stage, the PSA, and the grade, as well as how Jim's numbers compared.

	Stage	PSA	Grade
Ideal	T0	Below 4	2
Signals problems	T1	Over 4	3+
Life-threatening / high-risk	T3–T4	Over 20	Over 7
Jim	**T3**	**39.5**	**8**

Knowing the grade and stage of your prostate cancer helps you understand its state and its potential for future growth and spread. Keep in mind, however, that no detection and measurement system is foolproof. You must keep track of your own grade, stage, and PSA because, even though the doctors understand the numbers and letters better than you, they can make mistakes or misread your chart (or have the wrong chart pulled). The more knowledgeable you are about the state of your illness, the more empowered you are to take an active role in your own treatment.

GOING TO SEE THE DOCTORS

In the middle of difficulty lies opportunity.

—Albert Einstein

Our next step was to visit specialists who could give us more specific answers to the hundreds of questions running through our minds. Often it may take months to get in to see a top doctor who is in great demand. I learned a good trick early on: Take the first available appointment, and then gently inquire about the possibility of getting an earlier one. This can sometimes move up an appointment by days, weeks, and, in some cases, months. Another way to obtain an early appointment is to ask your primary care doctor to help you arrange meetings with specialists. The informal but powerful network of doctors and nurses who can work on your behalf is crucial to securing access to some of the better doctors. Dr. Chun's office was very helpful in getting us an appointment with Dr. Chinn, a well-respected urologist, within a week of Jim's initial test results.

Specialists can offer you a great deal of information about your disease and the complexities associated with it. We found that by preparing questions ahead of time, we were able to get the most out of each doctor. During the actual visit, we also wrote down answers to our questions and notes that we could review later. This worked well for us because, although we thought we were listening closely at the time, we probably weren't taking that much in. There were so many thoughts swirling around in our heads as the doctor was speaking, and so many new terms to absorb, that it helped us to write things down. Not only will writing give you a detailed record of your visits, but it will also help when you go to look up information in medical reference books. Anything you can do to take charge of your health care will be invaluable to you in the long run.

The Urologist

The urologist's office was located next door to the hospital. Hospitals cure people. Jim needed to be cured, so it seemed comforting to be near a hospital. Even so, it was uncomfortable and unfamiliar for us to be in places with "sick" people.

As we entered Dr. Chinn's office, we saw several men in their seventies. In the waiting room there was literature placed methodically by each set of chairs. Brochures, magazine headlines, videos—prostate cancer was everywhere, hitting us right between the eyes. There was nowhere to hide from it.

Within ten minutes the nurse called out Jim's name. It was business as usual at the busy medical office. But for us this was not an everyday event, it was one of the defining moments in our lives. Jim and I were on the brink of discovering our next steps in life, the future of Jim's health, the strength of our resolve and our love. There was no turning back time: Cancer was in our life and places such as this office, and places where cancer is an accepted reality would become new homes for us. We could no longer avoid the cold, bare facts. We would have to face cancer head-on.

The nurse directed us toward a long, narrow hallway and into Dr. Chinn's private office. It was a sparse, windowless room, quite small, with a desk, bookshelves, and two simple chairs for visitors. The office seemed as barren as we felt. By contrast, Dr. Chinn had a friendly manner that made us feel welcome in the tight quarters. However, the confined air in the room seemed as though it was pressurized at five hundred pounds per square inch. Dr. Chinn appeared to be visibly surprised at Jim's healthy and vibrant appearance. I sensed he was reflecting to himself, "This guy is not much older than me—so young to have such advanced prostate cancer. It could be tough for this couple to accept the news."

Dr. Chinn left us briefly to retrieve Jim's file, and we both sat there in fear of what we would learn next. My heart was beating furiously, and I could feel myself beginning to perspire. I reached over for Jim's hand, and it, too, was warm. We were both processing our nervous energy and emitting heat like crazy in that tiny office. Jim was glancing around at the cancer materials and books, trying to maintain his composure. The doctor returned to two frightened individuals who looked like deer in headlights, waiting to be hit. Only the blow would not come from a car; it would come from this kind doctor's mouth. His words could be as swift and devastating as a speeding car barreling directly into us. Neither of us felt ready to take the full impact of the news.

As Dr. Chinn opened the file, there was a pause while he reviewed the test results. He already knew Jim had advanced prostate cancer, the tests were dire in regard to the full extent of his condition. Now he would have to deliver the bad news. The doctor spoke in a soft, low tone that was calming and assured. This made hearing the words less abrasive, but the message was as devastating as any two words can be—"inoperable cancer."

Instantly, the office felt like it was closing in on me. I wanted to run. As Dr. Chinn spoke, my heart felt a sharp pain; it was physically aching and hurt. My pulse raced, and I struggled to control myself because of Jim. How he must have been feeling right then. He already felt confused and anxious from knowing it was serious.

Dr. Chinn told us that we could explore many options, but one thing was certain: Jim's cancer was too advanced for surgery. More than once during the conversation, he told Jim how surprised he was that Jim had such a serious case of the disease. But Dr. Chinn also offered the beginnings of a treatment plan, something Jim could do immediately, fight against cancer. He told Jim that he could start hormone therapy that very day.

> "Dr. Chinn, based on my test results, what would you do if you were me?" Jim asked.
>
> "It really depends on you," Dr. Chinn calmly replied. "There are hormone-therapy treatments like Lupron and Casodex, but they have side effects that some men cannot handle well. Some cancers continue to grow even with these drugs, because they grow independently of testosterone. However, in most cases, testosterone fuels the cancer, and we need to starve the cancer cells from their source of it."
>
> "You mean one of your recommended options is for me to prevent my body from producing testosterone?"
>
> "Yes, and there are two primary ways to do this. One way is through surgical castration; the other is through hormone therapy, whereby we literally shut down your body's ability to produce testosterone."

This was almost unimaginable to me. The idea of a man having his testicles removed—how awful. Here we were sitting in a doctor's office, learning that the hormones that make a man a man were actually killing Jim. The testosterone required by any man to be strong, vibrant, and sexually active actually cause this cancer to grow. Jim was in a life-and-death situation, and now we understood there would be trade-offs on the quality of our life together. Who could imagine giving up the ability to have sex? Was Jim worried about what would happen to our relationship? Would I still love him?

For me, as Jim's partner and soul mate, the decision was easy. I'd rather have Jim, the person, in my life than Jim, the "man," with a body full of deadly testosterone. At moments like this I began to understand the discussions common in the medical community about quality of life and the side effects of treatment.

While we still were not sure of Jim's treatment plan, there was one thing we were sure of: We weren't going to leave the doctor's office without doing something. With a sense of desperation and hope, we asked Dr. Chinn what Jim should do to start to cure this dreadful disease. We needed help and wanted a clear solution, even though we could tell there wasn't one. There were only choices, not definitive answers.

We knew right then we had to do whatever it would take, and wanted to begin as soon as possible.

"I can give you a shot today," said Dr. Chinn. "However, be aware, your sexual performance will be affected almost immediately. At first you'll have a short boost in sexual performance, but it will probably deteriorate over the following couple of weeks or months. Other potential side effects are, you'll probably gain weight, as much as 10 to 15 pounds, plus your breasts may grow, and you could lose your body hair."

Because of my naiveté and lack of experience with cancer drugs, I thought they were supposed to take away your problems, not burden you with more. This was awful, and there was no way to sugarcoat the message—it was not going down easily. I was just sitting there, dumbfounded. What a terrible drug, I kept thinking. Weren't there any better drugs?

"Are there any other options?" I asked. "What else can we do?"
"Well," said Dr. Chinn, "right now there really aren't many options, but there are advances happening all the time in

prostate cancer treatment. If you want, you can contact other major prostate-cancer centers to see what they are doing and to ask for their recommended treatment plan. Also, I suggest you go see our resident oncologist and get his opinion. He's highly respected and can give you another perspective on your condition."

"I want to be aggressive in treating my cancer," Jim replied.

This was the first time he had said "my cancer." He was moving from denying to accepting that he, Jim Miller, really had cancer and there was nowhere to run from it.

"I am not just going to accept the status quo and sit back and let this cancer grow and potentially kill me."

Dr. Chinn responded, "There is a great reference guide that I use myself and also recommend to all of my prostate-cancer patients, *The ABCs of Prostate Cancer*. If you're willing to travel to get a second opinion, I recommend that you go to the cancer clinic at the University of California at San Francisco [UCSF]. From my perspective, the leading researchers on prostate cancer are at UCSF; MD Anderson, in Houston; Seattle Medical Center; and Harvard Medical Center, in Boston. Each has its own perspective, so if you really want to explore other options, those would be the places to go. I was fortunate enough to work with Dr. Stamie at UCSF, and I would be more than happy to put you in touch with him. But before you go, I recommend you go locally and see Dr. Chung, a very well-respected oncologist here in Honolulu.

"These sound like some good next steps," Jim offered, "Thank you, Dr. Chinn. I'll start with the Lupron shot today and figure out where we go from here."

Taking the First Steps

There we were in a windowless, stuffy room, attempting to start our journey of active healing and curing. The pressure was building as we realized this was a journey we would be mapping out ourselves. Yes, the doctors were helpful, but they were not us, they were not the person or the family going through the experience. They were the directors at a theater, and we were the actors on stage. They had to be detached and directive with their advice to remain objective. We were the ones with the feelings. The ones who were ultimately responsible for our choices, the performers of our own lives and destiny. It was as though we were headed up a massive mountain with no road map. The doctors were there to act as guardrails, so we didn't drive off the edge, but they couldn't tell us the proven route up the mountain, only that we had to go over the top to reach the safety of a healthy life on the other side.

It seemed like a nonevent as Jim went into a treatment room we had passed earlier. However, this was not a simple shot Jim was getting—this was our first significant step towards giving his body the support it needed to fight the cancer. Perhaps we really could control the uncontrollable, I thought optimistically. He took off his shirt and I sat with him, holding his hand.

With his first Lupron shot, we started a more than four-year journey without much fanfare. Who would have known then that the journey would take us thousands of miles from home and span over a thousand days?

Our daily lives changed dramatically from that point on. Talk about a disorienting dilemma that changes your life! Suddenly, health becomes a major obsession. Once you find yourself needing serious health care, you are absorbed by spending hours at the doctor's office and by researching the vast amount of information you need to make the right choices. You invest incredible amounts of time you never knew you had. Health care is big business in our country, and the patient's huge decision is how to use his precious resources of time and money. As we learned, you must be prepared to expend personal energy on all aspects of the patient's health care.

The visit to the next specialist, the oncologist, demonstrated the costs of the visits. The visit costs seemed to keep rising as we saw doctors with higher and higher degrees of specialization. However—big business or not—we needed to do everything in our power to get Jim healed and cured. The business side of it just seems to make it all too impersonal and shallow, but it is always there in the background. For others who do not have the financial means to pay for these services, there are many outreach programs. Hospitals offer financial aid, and there are even organizations and grants in various communities to help those in need through this experience. A short list is referenced in the resources section in the appendix.

We took Doctor Chinn's advice and went to see the oncologist, Dr. Chung. Concurrently, we started on our quest to get appointments and learn from some of the best cancer-treatment facilities. What we found in trying to heal Jim's disease was that there was no immediate fix; it was going to take years. We were not involved with a sprint for life here, but with a marathon to recovery and healing.

The Oncologist

Although we had heard that surgery was not an option for Jim, somehow we hoped that would be the silver bullet. Why not just "go in, cut it out, and get rid of the cancer all at once?" This seemed the simplest and easiest solution.

As we went to Dr. Chung's office, we felt better prepared to discuss the severity of Jim's illness. What we were not prepared for was seeing so many other "dying" people in his office. It is hard to describe, but the feeling that people were fading away gave the office an aura that was eerie and macabre. When we entered the small office, only two other patients were there. From their appearance, they were well into the later stages of their illness. The signs included emaciation, limited hair, the need for a wheelchair, and occasional gasps and moans of pain. The despair and suffering in the room was overwhelming.

One of the patients was an older gentleman who sat quietly in his wheelchair. After a few minutes, I noticed he was in conversation with a younger woman, who appeared to be his loving daughter. She reached over to him and gently placed her hands on his frail body. She was reaching out to him, offering to run her hands over his emaciated body. She rubbed him ever so gently. While she rubbed, you could see the tears well up in her eyes, but he was grimacing—the trade-off between pain and attention left him no choice.

The other patient was an elderly woman, in need of serious care. She had a walker and a full-time nurse by her side. As the women sat there, I felt that the office space was a physical extension of her reality. The waiting room was a pale pink, like the pallor of the elderly woman's lips, with barely enough blood circulating in them to keep them flushed and full of life. The entire place epitomized impending death—the color, the smell, the aura.

The visit with Dr. Chung was not much better than the one with Dr. Chinn, not because of the doctor himself, but because of the message he had for us. We soon realized we had come for a conversation, not an exam. We were learning that there are times when doctors will merely counsel you and not perform tests, exams, or prescribe any drugs. For us, this was a first. Dr. Chung was tall and had an air of confidence, so when he spoke you knew he was comfortable with the subject of cancer, treatment, and dying. That ease made it a little less difficult to bear, but still the visit was extremely depressing. He informed us unequivocally that surgery was not a viable option. Since the disease had spread beyond the prostate, the doctors could not get "the margins" needed to get all the cancer out.

It was there that we learned that the five-year survival rate for someone with Jim's condition was about 15 to 20 percent. This meant around 80 percent of the people diagnosed with prostate cancer at this grade, stage, and PSA count were dead within five years because of prostate cancer or some other cause. This was a serious blow, and the gravity of the situation struck us to the core.

Dr. Chung told us that there was a patient on Kauai that had a similar PSA level as Jim. "He used hormone therapy and is still alive after over ten years," Dr. Chung said. But he told us many people with levels so severe had died. He looked at Jim kindly. "Enjoy the time you have left. The cancer has advanced so far at such an early age. Plus, the cancer is very aggressive."

We knew the doctor dealt with this reality every day, and, in a way, one had to respect his commitment to assist so many patients who he would be leading from life to death.

However, that was no comfort to us. We were devastated by the news but too much in shock to realize it at that moment. Bodies and souls work together in such crises in life. When one is absolutely blown out of the water, the other tries to rise to the occasion. We remained there in the office and were able to continue without getting overly emotional. Reflecting on this now, it is utterly amazing to think we could initially cope with even the direst news. This type of experience still causes an ache in my heart, even years later. Like a scar, it may heal, but the memory of the trauma is still there.

Dr. Chung recommended radiation as an additional treatment to the hormone therapy, however he candidly told us radiation may not work. If it did not work, the only other treatment would be to participate in clinical trials; however, he was not keen about this option. Such trials are the testing of experimental drugs and are normally done in three phases, each successive phase involving a larger number of people. Going through clinical trials would take a lot of effort, and the data to date had not shown any real results. He also felt that clinical trials have unknown risks, including a dramatic impact on quality of life, and even death.

In addition to wanting more information on hormone therapy, we were curious about alternative medicine. Our questions on this topic were met with a lukewarm response. Dr. Chung did not elaborate much on the subject, but we could tell he believed strongly that the Western approach to treating cancer made the most sense. On the other hand, he did not discourage us from seeing other doctors to get additional opinions. He knew we were still seeking and were not satisfied. It was clear we expected more and wanted more alternatives.

How Did I Get Prostate Cancer?

One of our most profound, unanswerable questions during this experience with cancer was "How?" We asked Dr. Chung for his theory on how Jim could have developed prostate cancer. The doctor didn't know, and he believed that current medical research could offer no answers. There are many theories about how cancer develops—from genetic flaws, damaged cells, viruses, exposure to toxins, having a vasectomy, and others—but no definitive conclusion. What we did learn at Dr. Chinn's office was *virtually all men get prostate cancer* at some point in their lives if they live long enough.

This may sound like a radical statement. The reason virtually all men get prostate cancer is not fully understood, but the likelihood of a serious prostate condition increases with age. In many cases, the disease grows so slowly that there is no impact on the man's health. Some prostate cancer cells take over four years to double. To be affected, the average man would need in excess of a million cancer cells growing and doubling much more rapidly than once every year. Autopsy studies have revealed that invasive prostate cancer is present in 40 percent of men over fifty years old, and this statistic increases with age. However, it is estimated that only 8 percent of prostate cancers will become significant in a man's lifetime, and roughly 3 percent of men will die from prostate cancer.

Seeking Additional Information

After our visit to the oncologist, we were immensely saddened and, at the same time, more committed than ever to fight the cancer. We were not just going to accept the status quo. This was just not acceptable to us. This was about Jim's life.

Jim was not ready to share his condition with anyone other than me until he had a better understanding of what he would be doing now that he was ill. We wanted to be open about the situation with our family, especially our children. Jim felt we needed to learn more for ourselves before we shared details with anyone. This gave him time to cope with having to maintain the role of father while accepting the reality of the situation. It was an important time for Jim to gather his composure before publicly sharing his situation. It was vital he do this on his terms.

We agreed that I would spend the day learning as much as possible about prostate cancer. I placed calls to Jim's insurance company, the human resources office at his company, the doctor's office, the National Institute of Health, and many others. The morning hours flew by without much progress. We were on a quest to discover as much as possible. I learned there was an endless amount of things we didn't know. Not only were there the complex, detailed medical facts to absorb, but all the games played between the drug companies, insurance companies, and the medical community. My goal was to fulfill my commitment of love for Jim, to help the two of us learn about the very best options for him.

Part of my frantic quest was to find out the names and numbers of the potentially best doctors in their respective fields. This was no small feat, but I did find a resource called *The Best Doctors in America*, offered by Best Doctors Worldwide Healthcare Service, that lists U.S. doctors' top choices, the crème de la crème. This organization creates a database of their names, covering all types of doctors, well beyond oncologists and urologists. The service is a great starting point for finding a superior doctor. A patient- care coordinator helped me navigate the extensive database and cull the file to five or so potential doctors.

In the afternoon, before Jim came home from the office, I went to three bookstores, two local and one national chain, and bought up every book on cancer and prostate cancer. Standing in front of the medical section at the national chain bookstore I was surprised to see how few books about cancer there were on the shelves. There was only one book specifically about prostate cancer, and I bought it. It was an uncomfortable feeling—the first time in my life buying books about cancer. Was the person to my right looking at me quizically because I was in the medical books section, wondering what was wrong with me, or just casually looking around? Now perfect strangers, people outside our doctors' world, were going to know or suspect that someone I knew had prostate cancer. It was no longer our secret, and it made me feel weak and vulnerable. Jim and I were not used to feeling this exposure.

Interestingly, there were not many books dedicated to prostate cancer in the major bookstores. Maybe it's just a sign of where we are as a society—repressing such a personal sexual disease, an uncomfortable issue. I found information in disparate places, and it took a lot of effort to bring it all together and eventually synthesize it into a treatment and healing plan. I did find a few books through referrals and research we both really liked, such as *The ABCs of Prostate Cancer* by Joseph Oesterling, M.D., and Mark Moyad, M.P.H.; *50 Essential Things to Do When the Doctor Says It's Cancer* by Greg Anderson, and *Journey Into Healing* by Deepak Chopra, M.D.

The Internet is a powerful tool. Some websites we visited included www.prostatecancer.com and www.cancer.org.

Getting a Second Opinion

Jim's test results were tough to accept, and we found ourselves defying them even though I had read all the material we could get our hands on about prostate cancer and various treatments. We were also not satisfied with the information we received from the first three doctors, not because they were not solid doctors, but because we were on a quest for a deeper knowledge of what was happening to Jim. We wanted more; we hoped for more; we could not just settle for information we learned initially. So we decided that it was up to us to create an individual healing plan for Jim, based on what was right for us.

Jim and I believe success in life comes from expecting more from yourself. In the case of cancer, we believed in expecting more from Jim's body, more from the doctors, and more from our spirit as human beings. Cancer drives that lesson home in a big way. For us, it was a fundamental principle of living. As writer Somerset Maugham wrote, "It's a funny thing about life, if you refuse to accept anything but the best, you often get it."

Many people have negative things occur in their lives and blame others, or they run away from the situation. Jim and I had never been known to take the easy way out, and we were not about to do it now. We were committed to doing everything in our power to fight this—in every way possible.

People who say, "Get a second opinion," are absolutely right. In the field of prostate cancer treatment, there are myriad options and combination therapies, and we owed it to ourselves—and to Jim's life—to learn about all of them. We researched the best cancer treatment facilities in the United States, and along with input from Dr. Chinn, decided that the UCSF Cancer Center seemed like the best choice, as it is one of the leading cancer research institutions and treatment facilities in the country. Also, a colleague of Jim's, who had successfully been treated for prostate cancer at UCSF, gave us the name of his doctor. We opted to visit a well-known surgeon and close colleague of the UCSF doctors, Dr. Skinner, at the University of California at Los Angeles (UCLA).

UCSF Cancer Center

We called the clinic at UCSF and found out it would take more than two months to get in for an initial visit. This would have been fine if we had been waiting for furniture to be delivered, but it was not an acceptable amount of time to wait while Jim's life was at stake. The more we read about cancer, the more we understood that time was of the essence. I believed our best course of action was to "sell" ourselves to these doctors. We had to let them know how dedicated we were to the process of Jim's healing and how much we needed to see them as soon as possible. So we drafted a letter to the doctor we wanted to see at UCSF.

Below is the letter we used to secure an appointment, which you may want to use as a sample.

Peter Carroll, M.D.
UCSF
Dept. of Urology/Oncology
2300 Sutter St. Suite 205
San Francisco, Ca. 94115

Dear Dr. Carroll,

Please accept this letter as a request to see you at your earliest available time. Also, please consider that time is of the essence in treating my particular case of prostate cancer. You have been referred to us by one of your former patients and our current urologist in Hawaii. Additionally, our primary-care physician has recommended your group as being one of the best in the country for the treatment of prostate cancer.

The cancer was detected before I turned fifty, and I already have PSA of 39. We have had completed PSA tests, a biopsy, an MRI, and computed tomography, and have the results available for your review. We will come for an office visit and for full treatment as your schedule permits. We have the flexibility and commitment to getting the best possible treatment. At this time, our primary-care physician is recommending that we proceed with treatment as soon as possible.

I am in excellent physical shape, except for the cancer, which is either in stage C or stage D. Last week I called to schedule an appointment, and your assistant was kind enough to return the call. I hope this note will make you aware of the degree of my illness, my desire to seek your advice, and my commitment to being the most dedicated patient possible.

Thank you for your consideration in advance. I look forward to meeting you and working through this challenge together.

Respectfully yours,

Jim Miller

We wrote the letter for Jim while at graduate school. I was very busy because school was ending in two months. However, the pressure of final exams and completed papers was nothing compared to what I was feeling about Jim, his illness, and our lives. No one in my class knew of my situation. Quite frankly, it was easier that way: I did not need to expend any energy explaining what was going on and why I was feeling overwhelmed. Before cancer, it had been so important for me to get my Masters; now it seemed unimportant. Jim and I decided the right thing for me was to continue and complete what I had started rather than use cancer as an excuse to take the easy way out. Cancer was changing our lives, but it was not stopping us—we were going to make it through this, and we would emerge stronger individuals.

The letter turned out to be one of our best strategies for securing top medical advice. We were able to see the doctors at UCSF within three weeks. This was a significant boost for us, because it made us feel empowered and in charge of Jim's treatment.

On our first morning in San Francisco, we woke up early and went for a run along the Embarcadero. It was a cool morning, like most in San Francisco, and the water on the bay resembled a flat sheet fitted tightly on a bed—no ripples, no wrinkles, just flat.

Perfect for us at that moment, calming and energizing at the same time. We talked about what our meeting would be like while we were jogging along, even though we had no idea what we were getting into at UCSF. We thought a meeting with Dr. Carroll would be helpful to us no matter what our future decisions would be, and that made us feel good. We were not being helpless victims, but active participants in dealing with cancer.

Upon entering the UCSF building, we could tell this place was different from where we had been before. It was known as a dedicated cancer-treatment facility, and the entire building seemed to be designed specifically for people with cancer. Ahead of us was a long hallway with a row of windows on one side that looked out onto a beautiful English-garden courtyard. There was a peace to the garden that filled the hallway with a sense of universal hope and brightness. To me, it represented the beauty that continues to exist around us even in our darkest hours. For the few moments that we were there, we felt the positive energy of life and the vitality of the flowers.

In the elevator we noticed that the floors were laid out according to the type of cancer, and it was eye-opening to realize the scope and variety of cancers that exist. Our doctor's office was on the third floor. By the time we arrived, almost all the waiting room chairs were taken. Jim asked a gentleman to move, enabling us to sit next to each other. We wanted to be near each other because it made us feel more comfortable and secure. The chairs were occupied mostly by older men of different ethnic and social backgrounds. Most were there alone, but there was one homosexual couple. It was obvious that this disease knew no demographic boundaries.

We had brought Jim's X-rays with us on the plane, and his file had been sent directly from the urologist's office in Hawaii. Before coming, we made sure to confirm that the file had arrived at UCSF, to avoid any hassles. This is always a good precaution to take, because files do not always get sent on time and can get lost en route. Securing this appointment at UCSF was tough enough; therefore, we wanted to make absolutely sure the doctors had all the information at their fingertips, so they could give us the most informed advice.

Finally, we were face to face with Dr. Carroll. We were immediately comfortable with his demeanor, approach, and style. He told us that Jim would be seeing three doctors that day and would be free to ask the same or different questions of any of them. He explained that they each had their own area of expertise in prostate cancer. He, himself, was a surgeon, Dr. Phillips was the head of radiation oncology, and Dr. Small specialized in acute advanced disease. The interdisciplinary approach of determining which treatment options would be best for Jim was fantastic, informative, and from what we knew of other facilities, unconventional. It was refreshing, and gave us a sense of trust and openness. It was obvious that there was a mutual respect at UCSF for multiple disciplines and innovative thinking. Based on our experience in business, we knew that this was the best way to get increased effectiveness and a positive outcome. If it worked in business, it made sense to us that it would work just as well in a hospital setting.

First, Dr. Carroll examined Jim, giving him a DRE, during which I left the room. Upon my return, the doctor confirmed all the data we had so far indicating a large tumor and a serious problem. From his perspective, surgery was not a desirable option, and he would not recommend it. We would need to see Dr. Phillips, of radiation oncology, for his expert opinion on radiation therapy; Dr. Carroll suspected such a treatment might be our most logical option.

We learned from our visit with Dr. Phillips that he was winding down his career as chair of the department and would retire soon. He was very up-front and assured us that Dr. Roach, who was due back from vacation in two weeks, would become our radiation oncologist. His opinion of Jim's condition was that a combination of aggressive radiation with hormone therapy would be the preferred method of treatment. He answered all of our questions about treatment timing, side effects, and the pros and cons of other options. He never rushed us, and we felt he was genuinely interested in Jim's well-being, even though he was retiring. He told us that Dr. Roach would give us more details of the full, recommended treatment plan after he examined all of the files. Dr. Phillips did give some specifics that made us feel more confident about our next steps. For example, UCSF does 3-D conformal radiation, which allows them to directly target the radiation dosage and treatment to very specific parts of the body. (Not all hospitals have the equipment to do this.) Additionally, they were committed to radiating the pelvic and surrounding area because Jim had shown positive test results for cancer outside of the prostate.

Because Jim had a large tumor, they wanted to wait a few months to see if it would shrink from the hormone therapy and other drugs he was taking. Their goal was for the tumor to be completely unpalpable during a DRE before starting radiation. This approach made sense to us. One other question we had was about seed implants because they seemed so targeted. Seed implants are a form of radiation treatment, in which radioactive materials are placed directly into a cancer-affected organ with the intent of destroying the malignancy. Dr. Phillips informed us that because Jim's cancer was in both seminal vesicles and his pelvis, the seeds would not be able to work effectively. Making sure the seeds are placed properly is critical, and they work well if the cancer is contained within the prostate.

We expressed our desire to have Jim cured to Dr. Phillips, and asked him if he thought this possible despite Jim's advanced condition. Dr. Phillips was exceedingly cautious and told us that it depended on a number of factors, like how Jim's cancer responded to the hormone treatment over time, the level of radiation he would receive, how the PSA responded after radiation, and Jim's tolerance to radiation and the other treatments. We desperately wanted Jim to be cured by these treatments, and we already knew that hormone and chemotherapy alone would only control the disease, not cure it. From Dr. Phillips, we wanted to know that it could be cured.

Dr. Small's consultation was an informative and encouraging part of our visit—and very frightening. He managed cancer patients who were undergoing alternative clinical trial experiments. This was a man we never wanted to meet again professionally. (Socially he seemed wonderful but as a patient he was a "last hope" doctor.) He was there for those patients who had exhausted all other options. Jim did not need him yet, and hopefully never would. Dr. Small's manner was serious, but he also gave us hope that there was a safety net of future trials and research available if Jim's initial treatment plan did not work.

After the three consultations, the doctors left us alone for half an hour. This let us absorb all we had heard and discuss our feelings in private. No doubt, the doctors needed a chance to discuss Jim's case among themselves. Afterward, all three sat down with us for our final consultation. They did an amazing job. In less than a day, we felt we had a real plan for treating Jim. They integrated their expertise, answered all our questions, and left us feeling confidant that UCSF could give Jim the best chance for full recovery. Our treatment journey, which had started in Hawaii, was evolving into a plan that was real and positive.

Later, when we reflected on our visit, we felt that the fundamental strength of UCSF was the involvement of multiple doctors of diverse expertise and their collaborative approach. First, they were acting as a team, and our business experience had taught us that teams almost always perform better than individuals. Second, the fact that the doctors were from multiple disciplines—surgery, research, and radiology—made us more comfortable with their collaborative recommendations. We felt we were getting the benefit of a medical check-and-balance system, just as the executive, congressional, and judiciary branches of our government balance power and decision making.

DEALING WITH EMOTIONS

We cannot escape fear. We can only transform it into a companion that accompanies us on all our adventures.

—Susan Jeffers

The night we returned home to Hawaii from our first visit to the urologist, it was impossible to sleep. Jim and I tossed and turned most of the night, rolling over and asking if the other was awake—the answer was yes. Jim rose early as usual, around 4:00 A.M. Our breakfast was as gray as a storm-filled sky, neither of us wanting to talk about the cancer yet. Both of us were trying to understand how to communicate with each other. We knew Jim had cancer. What was going to change? From the moment it was clear the tests were accurate, cancer was in our lives. We were now on a new path, one that forced us to examine what was really important in life. At morning breakfast, most important was to be together, to look into each other's eyes with love and fear, and just be. Life was going to be different and unpredictable. There were few words when Jim left for work as I cried.

What Is Relevant Changes

How quickly life can change in a matter of just a couple of weeks. I had been in the closing phase of a buying a business and licensing a world-class brand in Hawaii, and Jim had been in the thick of it with his career. We were two souls racing through life, thinking we were living when we were actually letting it pass us by; we were moving too fast to take time to notice the subtleties of being a human being. What mattered most to us in life was work; what others thought about who we were as people, parents, and citizens; and still more work. Now, much of this seemed insignificant and irrelevant to the challenge we were handed.

When we first found out about the cancer, Jim wanted to quit his job outright. Luckily, logic took over, and he did not. The idea of changing his focus from work to working on being totally well seemed attractive at first. However, we soon realized one doesn't act impulsively with a life-threatening disease. Jim needed to maintain his health insurance. Work serves as a way to cope in the beginning, because it distracts you with the myriad details that demand your attention, and because it provides that familiar sense of rhythm and continuity to your life. It also fills up the "white space," the time between doctor visits and treatments, with something to think about other than cancer. If you're not careful during these times, you could let your mind go, you could get yourself all upset, scared to death, and miserable about the situation at hand. It's important to allow for some self-exploration and reflection; however, days of it at a time can cause mild or severe depression.

Once, when we left a doctor's office, I noticed a small sign, CANCER RESOURCE CENTER. Odd—probably a month earlier I would have passed by the sign without even noticing. All of a sudden the idea of relevancy had a whole new meaning. When you find yourself in a life-threatening crisis, you suddenly relate deeply to certain events, signs, conversations, and newspaper articles with a real desire to comprehend what is being said since they are relevant to your very existence. Jim and I were learning about having compassion for others who are in a wide variety of struggles for life and well-being. The human condition was a concept we had never fully embraced before. The world is so full of suffering and disease—it is one of life's heartbreaking realities. Disease touches everyone, no matter who they are or where they live. The lesson in life may be one of learning to be more understanding of each other, and learning we all need help, love, and healing in one way or another at some point in our lives.

Could I Die?

Approach each new problem not with a view of finding what you hope will be there, but to get the truth, the realities that must be grappled with. You may not like what you find. In that case, you are entitled to try to change it.

—Bernard M. Baruch

As one's understanding of their illness moves from denial to acceptance, there is a painful effect. One awakens to the reality of how terrible the situation really is and how grim the statistics really are. We read reports that indicated Jim's life expectancy after five years would be below 20 percent. We had also been told that if the cancer continued to grow at the same rapid pace, Jim could lose his life in only two to three years. This was not something we were eager to believe, and we struggled to be honest with ourselves about what the future held. We tried to maintain hope so that we would not be totally debilitated; however, our fear was overwhelming at times. It was that formless, pervasive fear of the unknown that comes with facing a silent and hidden enemy. We weren't sure we could win this battle.

One Sunday, two weeks after the battery of test results confirmed the severity of Jim's illness, we finally allowed ourselves to think the unthinkable. We realized that this disease could very likely kill Jim. The reality hit us, as we've found with so many aspects of the cancer experience, when we least expected it.

It was a beautiful Hawaiian day. We had gone for a run in the morning, had been to church, and felt fabulous, but behind the perfect facade was profound uneasiness and sadness that we had suppressed by being busy and avoiding our real feelings. Our "busy-ness" took us to the Ala Moana Mall in Honolulu, where Jim bought me a beautiful navy jacket. We were feeling great as we left the store and walked to the parking lot. We got in the car, and as Jim started to pull out, we realized how precious that moment was—so present, so alive, so energized. It was a spectacular moment: We were so happy to be able to enjoy each other and the beauty of the world around us. How could this be at risk? How could this be temporary? The fear of losing this moment forever hit both of us at the same time. It was overwhelming, almost as if a cloud of darkness had come over our car. Jim started sobbing, "Please, please, Julia, don't let me die without my dignity. I want people to remember me like I am now."

In the back of my mind I knew he was thinking of himself as a sick, dying man, and the thought of it was too much for him to bear. It was not so much that Jim was afraid of dying; he was profoundly saddened by the speed of change and the end of something joyous. We both sobbed uncontrollably. Jim was crying so hard we had to pull off to the side of the road. Sadness filled our souls.

Depression

Learn to get in touch with the silence within yourself and know that everything in this life has a purpose.

—Elizabeth Kubler-Ross

Depression is a serious problem for men with prostate cancer and is common in American men over fifty years of age. This is an age when many men may first realize they are not immortal and thus reflect on their life and accomplishments, leading to feelings of doubt and regret. Declining health and sexual dysfunction may bring on feelings of gloom and despair. The diagnosis of prostate cancer can cause significant stress and may push someone with depressive tendencies into a full-blown depression.

There is a question in the medical community as to whether cancer can cause biochemical changes in the body that result in depression. Currently, there is no definitive answer. However, side effects from treatment may contribute to an overall depressive state. Surgery and radiation therapy can cause severe fatigue, and androgen withdrawal causes male menopause and is well known to trigger depression in some men.

Depression complicates the treatment of prostate cancer. Depressed men may believe that treatment is hopeless or feel that the side effects of treatment are just too much to bear. These feelings could lead them to delay seeking treatment until it is too late. Depressed men may not sleep well, and may forget to take their medication, eat properly, or otherwise take care of themselves. Whether we like to admit it or not, depression and anxiety are important problems for men with prostate cancer. Untreated, these problems cause psychological pain and suffering and can disrupt relations with family members and loved ones.

When someone first learns they have cancer, it is common to experience shock and disbelief. This is usually followed by a period of anxiety and depression, which is often mixed with anger. It is important to understand that this is a natural, though painful, progression of feelings, but you must get through them and reach the next stage of acceptance to be able to journey to recovery and wholeness.

Many cancer patients and loved ones have trouble sleeping through the night. I did, even though I was not the one undergoing treatment. Jim was exhausted from his treatments, yet he was able to sleep just fine. Insomnia exacerbates the stress caused by cancer, because both patient and family need all their strength to fight the disease. Some men will wake up every night between two and three in the morning and not resume sleep until around five. This dark time is usually temporary and resolves once the patient and his physician embark on a new treatment plan. Support of family and friends can speed the resolution of these symptoms.

There are many patients in whom the symptoms of anxiety, anger, and depression persist. A recent study by the Psychosocial Collaborative Oncology Group (PSYCOG) examined the emotional health of a group of 215 randomly selected adult cancer patients. They found that 53 percent were adjusting normally to the stress of their diseases. The remaining 47 percent had clinically apparent psychiatric problems. In 89 percent of the patients, these problems were in reaction to their disease and did not represent preexisting emotional illness. For close to two thirds of the 47 percent, the psychological problems were judged to be transient in nature. However, 13 percent of the patients had developed a major depression. The presence of pain made it much more likely that the patient would have significant depression and anxiety.

Jim went through a serious bout of depression right after the radiation treatments were over. From February through September, he had been single-mindedly pursuing activities that made him feel like he was fighting the disease. Whether it was acupuncture, radiation, or his support groups, he knew he was engaged body, mind, and soul in defeating the cancer. Once the daily radiation treatments were over, a time of anxious waiting began. We had prepared for battle, fought for months, and now we were going to have to wait and see if the outcome would lead to victory or defeat. It was not the sweet, sudden victory you can achieve in a game or a war, but a slow, worrisome progress that often appears to be fleeting. The initial major battle was over, but there would be more, and Jim was going to have to wait for the final outcome.

Depression creeps up on you as an individual and as a couple. At first you don't even notice it. You find yourself making excuses like, "I really don't want to go out tonight," or, "I'll wait and call the kids next week," or, "Mom and Dad have too many other things going on to call them." It enters your life quietly and changes you. For us it was subtle and it stayed for well over a year. We had thought that Jim would come off all treatments after one year, but our doctors felt he was physically tolerating the drugs well enough to continue treatment. Breast cancer studies had proven that women who continued treatment for two years had longer survival rates. Prostate cancer like breast cancer is a hormone-based cancer, and prolonged treatment would be advisable. The news was quite a blow to Jim and I. We had thought we were close to the top of our mountain of struggle, only to learn we still had a long way to go. Although we were grateful for how Jim's body was responding to the treatment, we were anxious to know if the treatment had worked. Jim's PSA scores were very promising, consistently below .002 in the first six months after radiation, so all indications were positive. Yet we still had to remain cautious.

Life moves on and you do what you have to do. For us, the decision to prolong treatment was easy to make because we felt we could not stop now. The journey was already draining, and we were feeling depressed, but we went on. And that is what you do, you move on one step at a time, making it up the mountain.

The good news is, there are many drugs available for depression, and your doctor will help determine the right choice. Jim worked through his depression without drugs, but looking back, I wonder whether we should have explored that option at certain times during his treatment and recovery. Listed below are several of the drugs available for depression and anxiety.

Selective Serotonin Reuptake Inhibitors (SSRIs)

SSRIs are drugs that enhance the effectiveness of brain waves by prolonging the presence of serotonin in the brain. There are four SSRIs currently available in the United States: Prozac (fluoxetine), Paxil (paroxetine), Zoloft (sertraline), and Celexa (citalopam).

New Antidepressants

These newer antidepressants differ from the SSRIs in that two other brain chemicals, norepinephrine and dopamine, are affected. It is not clear that any of the new drugs are superior to SSRIs.

- *Wellbutrin* (buproprion) appears to increase the effectiveness of dopamine.
- *Serzone* (nefazodone) acts on both norepinephrine and serotonin. This drug has proven in clinical trials to be as effective as the common SSRIs. However, it is much less likely than the SSRIs to cause a loss of sex drive, and it appears to alleviate insomnia and anxiety.

Drugs for Anxiety

Benzodiazepines include Valium, Librium, and Xanax. These cause rapid resolution of anxiety and panic and are useful sedatives and muscle relaxants. They are not well tolerated over the long term.

Relief From Hot Flashes

Megace is very effective in relieving hot flashes and can be associated with improved appetite. Unfortunately, Megace increases the risk of blood clots, particularly in the legs. Another huge potential drawback is that some prostate cancers have a mutation in their androgen receptor that causes Megace to increase the growth rate of the cancer.

Hot flashes are a common side effect of hormone therapy. Jim had as many as ten or more hot flashes a day when he was at the height of his radiation and hormone therapy. Sometimes the flash was so intense that he would literally be wet from head to toe. This seemed to happen in the evening while he was sleeping. Often he would need to move to another part of the bed, because the area where he lay was absolutely drenched. There was no rhyme or reason as to when or why he would get what we named "a flasher." They did seem less pronounced after acupuncture, but for Jim it was a small side effect and worth the inconvenience. He did not opt to explore drugs to treat hot flashes, because he felt already chock full of drugs, herbs, and vitamins.

THE FIRST THIRTY DAYS

Slow down and enjoy life. It's not only the scenery you miss by going too fast—you also miss the sense of where you are going and why.

—Eddie Cantor

The first thirty days of your cancer experience can be overwhelming, but it is wise to take time for yourself and process what is happening to you. You might have cancer, but it does not have you. You are still in control of your emotions, and you can take an active role in how you want to get through your journey.

To help contain the overwhelming number of things you need to do at this point, try mapping it all out on a calendar. This will help you feel more in control of the process, prevent you from missing important steps, and give you the sense that you are taking action about your situation. Below is an example of how you can create your first healing calendar. Add to it anything that applies to your personal situation, and use it as your guide through the tumultuous first month.

THE FIRST 30 DAYS

Doctors

- Determine your urologist, oncologist, and general practitioner
- Write down their contact info (phone and fax numbers, etc.) and office directions
- Check doctors' references.
- Consider using *The Best Doctors in America* to help make your decision.

Informing Family

- Determine your approach on how to tell them.
- Literally practice saying, "I have cancer," to prepare yourself.
- Be prepared for any type of reaction.

Insurance

- Confirm insurance coverage provided, and ask if there are any restrictions for particular doctors or institutions.
- Call insurance company to validate approval for doctor visits and treatment plan.

Work

- Check on your benefits at work.
- Contact human resources departmant and get the full insurance plan and disability details.

Gather Information

- Gather information from as many sources as possible to make the most informed decision (e.g., Internet, newsletters, cancer organizations and support groups).

Tests

- Confirm tests.
- Take all the tests each doctor recommends.
- Create a Prostate Cancer Healing journal or file, and be sure to keep your own records in it.

Explore New Options

- Explore joining a support group.
- Contact a nutritionist and/ or consider complementary medical options to enhance your treatment.

Treat Yourself

- Commit to stopping at least one thing you do that you really dislike.
- Take time each day to spiritually ask to be healed and cured.
- Take a full day to determine your treatment plan and what is most important to you.

Develop A Healing Action Plan

- Decide on your treatment plan.
- Write down your treatment plan.
- Commit to yourself that you are on the journey to healing and curing.

In the back of this book there is a "Sample Personal Medical Record," which contains the type of information you may need to track for an individual healing plan. By starting to document the details from the time of the initial diagnosis, you will save yourself a great deal of time and stress by having the key information in one place. Initially, this may seem overwhelming, but as you begin to learn more about what is happening, you will get better at managing your own healing process.

Be Sure You Know the Following

- Do you have any of the symptoms that were mentioned earlier in the book, such as painful urination, lower back pain, difficulty urinating, and so on?
- Have you been screened with a PSA test or a DRE? What are your test scores? Is there a potential problem?
- A doctor cannot diagnose prostate cancer from only an elevated PSA or PSAD levels. Have you scheduled additional tests?
- Additional tests might include the following: a digital rectal exam (DRE), transrectal ultrasonography (TRUS), an intravenous pyelogram, or a Cystoscopy. What are the results of these tests?
- What are the results of your biopsy? If the doctor is concerned there is cancer, he most likely will order a biopsy. A biopsy is the only foolproof way to know there is cancer.
- What is the stage and grade of your cancer?
- What are the results of all of your other tests? Be prepared to be the one who has this information to share with each doctor, as sometimes files are delayed, misplaced, or in the process of being updated.

While there are many other life events going on around you during this time—working, going out with friends, driving the kids around, food shopping, weddings, and so on—it is important to slow down. Try to take time for yourself to plan your healing journey. The more time you take to consider your options, the more comfortable you will be with your decision. This should give you the momentum to be totally committed to following through with your plan and knowing it is right for you.

Here are notes that Jim and I took during our first thirty days. You can see how his healing plan was beginning to unfold.

Our first priority was to determine the type of Western medical treatments we would pursue. After these decisions were made, we then considered alternative healing strategies, such as acupuncture, herbs, diet, and exercise.

NOTES / REMARKS DURING THE FIRST 30 DAYS

Documentation of conversations with our physician(s) or other health-care providers reminds us of important events, results of scans and X-rays, treatment opinions, etc.

3/6	Prognosis: serious illness. Dr. Chinn recommends hormone therapy. Briefly discussed aggressive alternative treatments. Potential recommendations for second opinion: Dr. Clayton Chung, Honolulu; UCSF LHRH hormone treatment and Casodex started.
3/9	Calls placed to UCSF head of dept. Dr. Carroll—high referral from *Best Doctors in America*. Call placed to establish initial contact.
3/14	Dr. Chinn refers Jim to Dr. Skinner a surgeon in addition to UCSF. Jim is feeling no side effects at this time. Letter written to Dr. Peter Carroll.
3/16	Dr. Peter Carroll's office–rescheduled appt. to 3/24 w/ Eric Small, Peter Carroll, and another doctor. Need to secure all test results/original copies (completed 3/18).
3/17	Dr. Clayton Chung—oncologist recommendation. Not favorable to surgery or progressive testing treatments, uncertain of benefits. It is critical to set an appointment one month after hormone therapy to see how PSA count is doing. The more dramatic the decline the better. From 39 to 8 or 9–lower is even better. God, please help us! Discussion of immunological testing. He is not interested: "Why recreate the wheel?" Insurance calls w/ H. H. Chun's office (primary physician). No need for consultative meeting.

	Preauthorizations—HMSA. After treatment recommended, call and tell them exact procedures, what will be covered and percentage.
3/18	Treatment and data discussion needed with Dr. Carroll—palliative or 3-D radiation, other immunological tests, timing, side effects, risks. Positive SF visit—Dr. Phillips, Dr. Carroll & Dr. Small. Dr. Roach will be our primary radial oncologist, and they will be our specialists, based on need. These are our guys—we like them and have decided to proceed with them
3/24	External & potentially internal radiation. Treatment to start after 4 mos. On hormones & Casodex, Lupron. Radiation requires daily visits plus preliminary planning/scanning visits prior daily to radiation therapy. 7/6 or later.
4/7	Dr. Chun revisit—LHRH shot & discussion of short-term disability; need to have PSA test done (completed). Follow-up note sent to Dr. Phillips & Dr. Roach regarding test results, 1.1, w/thank-you to Dr. Carroll & Dr. Small. Determined we will go to San Francisco for radiation treatment.

DETERMINING TREATMENT

Life shrinks or expands in proportion to one's courage.

—Anaïs Nin

In developing a treatment plan, you and your doctor will discuss the advantages and disadvantages of each treatment. The benefits of various treatments depend on how large the cancer has grown and how far it has spread—in other words, its stage. Your doctor must know enough about the behavior of your cancer and its exact location before he or she can recommend the best treatment for you. Proper and timely treatment can mean the difference between life and death, surgery versus radiation seeds, or a host of other consequences. If started at an early stage of prostate cancer, treatment can cure the disease. If treatment is started in a later stage, it can extend life and help relieve symptoms. Left untreated, prostate cancer can kill you.

Among American men with prostate cancer, thousands are alive today who exhibit no evidence of disease after five or more years since beginning treatment. This includes men who have undergone various types of treatments, such as surgery and radiation. Additionally, there are thousands of other American men who, while still showing evidence of the disease, continue to live comfortable and productive lives. As a result of new developments in treatment, men with prostate cancer are now living longer and with less discomfort and fewer treatment-related side effects. Advanced surgery techniques, like nerve sparring and seed implantation are leading to less permanent side effects and better quality of life.

One or more of the following methods may be recommended to you, depending on your condition and circumstances:

- Watchful waiting
- Surgery

- Radiation therapy (external beam 2-D/3-D or radioactive seeds)
- Cryosurgery
- Hormone therapy
- Chemotherapy

Each of these options will be described in the next few pages. However, before you and your doctor determine the proper treatment for you, a more detailed analysis of your condition is required. The method selected to treat prostate cancer depends on the stage of cancer, its speed of growth, and the age and general health of the patient. Treatment choice is based on how side effects might affect quality of life and other aspects of health. All these factors can and should be discussed thoroughly by you, your doctor, and your significant others.

Treatment Options

At the present time, certain recommendations are made more often than others for the treatment of each stage of prostate cancer. Your doctor will tell you the stage, grade, and other factors of your disease. The prostate cancer stages and common treatment choices are listed below. These treatments are described, first of all, based on your stage and, second, on the advantage and disadvantages of the treatment. As discussed earlier, the stage of the prostate cancer is crucial to determining the appropriate treatment. This information is meant only as a general guide. It is important to discuss this in depth with your doctor. Stages of prostate cancer range from stage A, the least advanced, to stage D, the most advanced.

Stage A

The tumor is located only within the prostate and is too small to be felt during a rectal examination. It causes no symptoms. If found at all, it is usually by chance, during surgery for a benign tumor or some other prostate disease, or by follow-up on screening tests that measure prostate-specific antigen.

Common treatments plans include surgery or radiation therapy. In some cases, no treatment at all may be needed. Instead, the cancer is simply watched ("watchful waiting") by your doctor, using digital rectal examinations and blood tests. Treatment may be started later if necessary.

Stage B

The tumor is still located only within the prostate but is large enough to be felt during a rectal examination. There are often no symptoms when a patient has this stage of prostate cancer.

Common treatment plans include surgery, cryosurgery, or radiation therapy. Cryosurgery involves the superfreezing of tissue in order to destroy it. It is used to treat malignant tumors and to control pain and bleeding. The freezing element is introduced through a probe, which has liquid nitrogen circulating through it. To destroy diseased tissue, it is cooled to below minus 20 degrees Celsius.

Stage C

The tumor has spread from the prostate to other nearby areas of the body. Difficulty urinating is a common symptom.

Common treatment plans include surgery, radiation therapy, or both. Hormone therapy or cryosurgery may be recommended.

Stage D

The tumor has spread to other parts of the body, most commonly the bones. Difficulty urinating, bone pain, weight loss, and fatigue are common symptoms.

Hormone therapy is usually the preferred treatment. Chemotherapy may be started at the same time or may be used later if hormone therapy does not work.

Specific treatment methods are described below. These were compiled from various *Prostate Forum* newsletters (www.prostateforum.com).

WATCHFUL WAITING

When the initial diagnosis is made, you may have a very low PSA level, or a very slow growth of prostate cancer. Virtually all men will get prostate cancer if they live long enough. It may be something that you can live with quite easily and that will not diminish your quality of life. This scenario is common in men in their seventies and older. The treatment here is simple: Every three to six months get a PSA blood test and monitor your PSA levels. If your cancer continues to grow slowly or not at all, your doctor will probably recommend continuing with this option.

ADVANTAGES: No change in your lifestyle; no surgery or other treatments required. There are no side effects from this activity. Only minimal time and energy is required to get regular PSA tests.

DISADVANTAGES: You must accept the fact that you will let your body exist with cancer growing inside it. You could possibly have a tumor that changes over time and becomes more virulent and, thus, more serious than your current case. You may forget to get monitored regularly and end up having a worse problem later.

REMOVAL OF THE PROSTATE BY SURGERY

Surgery can be used to remove cancer from the prostate and from nearby areas to which the cancer has spread. It is most often used during prostate cancer's early stages (stages A and B), when the cancer is located only within the prostate. Surgery may help prevent its further spread. If the cancer is small and located within the prostate, surgery may cure the disease.

One surgical procedure is called *perennial prostatectomy*. It involves removing the cancer through the perineum, the area between the scrotum and the anus. The entire prostate is removed, together with any nearby cancer.

Another procedure is called *retropubic prostatectomy*. It consists of removing the cancer through the lower abdomen. The entire prostate and nearby pelvic lymph nodes are removed.

ADVANTAGES: Prostatectomy is a one-time procedure that may cure prostate cancer in its early stages and may help extend life in the later stages. Surgery avoids the side effects and other problems of radiation therapy. Nerve sparing can limit side effects and still be successful in many cases

DISADVANTGES: Prostatectomy requires hospitalization and can produce unpleasant, permanent side effects, including impotence and incontinence (loss of urinary control). Impotence occurs in a high percentage of patients. Incontinence occurs in only a small percentage of patients but usually there is temporary incontinence after surgery. In recent years, however, the percentage of men with impotence following surgery has decreased because of a new nerve-sparing surgical technique.

CRYOSURGERY

The cryosurgery procedure works by injecting the tumor, and, if necessary, a limited area around it, with liquid nitrogen. This form of treatment is not as widely used as surgery and other treatments.

ADVANTAGES: This procedure kills all cells that are exposed to the liquid nitrogen and thereby eliminates the cancer cells.

DISADVANTAGES: Healthy cells are also killed in this procedure. If your urethra or bladder is exposed during surgery, you could have permanent difficulty and pain during urination.

RADIATION THERAPY

Radiation therapy uses high-energy rays to kill prostate cancer cells. Because the rays cannot be directed perfectly, they may damage cancer cells as well as healthy cells nearby. But if the dose of radiation is small and spread out over time, the healthy cells are able to recover and survive, and the cancer cells eventually die.

Usually, radiation therapy is given for prostate cancer that has not spread to distant areas of the body (stages A, B, and C). It is used to help prevent the cancer from spreading further. Like surgery, radiation works best when the cancer is contained in a small area. In early stages of prostate cancer, the therapy can cure the disease.

The treatment may be given for pain relief from prostate cancer that has spread to the bones (stage D).

There are two ways in which the high-energy rays can be delivered. In *external radiation therapy,* a machine delivers the radiation in brief sessions, usually one session each weekday for several weeks up to several months. There are two forms of radiation treatment given externally, two-dimensional and three-dimensional. The type of treatment available in your area depends on the equipment available to your radial oncologist. The benefit of the three-dimensional conformal radiation is that it can be more precisely targeted to the internal organs and the cancerous areas, allowing for higher doses to be administered.

In *internal radiation therapy,* the rays come from compounds placed inside the tumor or tumors. This type of treatment is exacting and can be used well when the patient's prostate cancer is confined to and around the prostate area. Internal radiation does not make the patient radioactive.

A newer and promising radiation treatment is *interstitial radiation therapy.* Here the rays come from tiny radioactive seeds inserted directly into the tumor. The seeds are inserted while the patient is under anesthesia; they are too small to cause discomfort. Since the seeds emit radiation where they are placed, it is important you have a doctor who is experienced in the placement of the seeds and who develops a plan for placement based on your specific cancer situation. The seeds release rays continually for about a year and remain in place for the rest of a person's life.

Another form of internal radiation is delivered by *injection* and is used for bone pain in stage D prostate cancer. Radioactive compounds go directly into the bone and may give dramatic pain relief to many patients.

ADVANTAGES: Radiation therapy can cure prostate cancer in its early stages and may help extend life in later stages. It rarely causes loss of urinary control, and it leads to impotence less frequently than does surgery. New injectable radioactive compounds, such as those containing radioactive strontium, may provide pain relief from cancer that has spread to the bone. These new compounds have fewer side effects than do the radioactive phosphorous compounds that have been available for many years.

DISADVANTAGES: Radiation therapy can cause a variety of side effects. Most are minor and disappear after the therapy is over.

The side effects include fatigue, skin reactions in the treated areas, frequent and painful urination, upset stomach, diarrhea, and rectal irritation or bleeding. Ongoing rectal bleeding may occur after treatments. When an external machine provides radiation therapy, it can cause the later development of impotence in some patients. Internal radiation therapy causes impotence less often, but may be associated with decreased white blood-cell and platelet counts.

HORMONE THERAPY

Hormone therapy is used to treat cancer that has spread beyond the prostate to areas such as the seminal vesicles, lymph nodes, lungs and/or bones (metastatic prostate cancer). Two types of hormone therapy can be used: 1) drugs that prevent the production or block the action of testosterone and other male hormones, or 2) surgical removal of the testicles, which make male hormones. Hormone therapy alone cannot cure prostate cancer. Instead, it slows the cancer's growth and reduces the size of the tumor or tumors.

Hormone therapy is most often used during advanced stages of cancer, when the disease has spread locally beyond the prostate (stage C) or into other areas of the body (stage D). This therapy helps extend life and relieve symptoms. When the cancer has spread beyond the prostate, complete surgical removal of the prostate is not common.

The primary strategy of hormone therapy is to decrease the production of testosterone by the testicles and the adrenal gland. Regardless of the method of hormone therapy, the decrease in testosterone can result in certain side effects. Antiandrogen and LHRH agonist (analog) drugs are available.

HORMONE THERAPY VIA DRUGS

Drugs involved in hormone therapy include *Lupron, Casodex,* and others.

ADVANTAGES: If administered in injection and pill form, the side effects of the treatment may not be permanent. There is no surgery with this type of treatment.

DISADVANTAGES: Side effects commonly include hot flashes, loss of sexual desire, and impotence. The cancer treatment can affect your sexual desire, ability to ejaculate or release semen, and ability to have erections. In many cases, the result is total impotence. You may develop prostate cancer that becomes hormone resistant after being treated for an extended period of time. Ongoing fatigue and weight gain are also common.

SURGICAL REMOVAL OF THE TESTICLES

An operation called *orchiectomy* removes the testicles, which produce most of the body's testosterone.

ADVANTAGES: Orchiectomy is an effective procedure that is relatively simple and performed only once. Often, the patient is given a local anesthetic and is allowed to go home the same day as surgery.

DISADVANTAGES: Orchiectomy is a surgical procedure, and many patients prefer a nonsurgical option if it will work as well. A good number of men also find it difficult to accept this type of surgery. Depending on the kind of anesthesia used, there may be special risks in certain types of patients. Orchiectomy may, in some cases, require hospitalization, and, of critical importance, it is not reversible.

ESTROGEN THERAPY

Another method is to administer a female hormone such as *estrogen* or *diethylstilbestrol* (DES) to help to mitigate the level of testosterone being produced. Female hormones reduce the production of testosterone by the testicles.

ADVANTAGES: Estrogen therapy is simple and only involves taking a pill. Unlike orchiectomy, the treatment does not include surgery, and its effects can be reversed.

DISADVANTAGES: Estrogen therapy produces various side effects. Estrogen can cause water retention, embarrassing breast growth and tenderness, and symptoms such as stomach upset, nausea, and vomiting. In addition, even low doses of estrogen may increase the risk of heart and blood-vessel problems.

These are the current treatments that are most common. There are, however new procedures and drugs being tested and introduced all the time. Be sure to ask your doctor about new and alternative treatments. See the charts at the back of this book for details on how test and treatment options overlap.

As you can see there are a wide variety of traditional Western medical options available to treat your prostate cancer. The tough part is for you and your doctor to determine the options that are right for you based on your goals, lifestyle, age, and condition.

Questions to Ask

Moving from diagnosis to a full understanding of your treatment options is not easy. Here are some questions to ask yourself to make sure you understand the range of options available to you. Based on the stage and grade of your cancer, what does your doctor recommend? What are the benefits and risks of each treatment?

- What is likelihood of survival rates after five years and longer?
- If you are seeing a general practitioner, has your doctor referred you to a specialist yet?
- Have you received a second opinion?
- Did the second opinion agree with the first opinion? If not, how will you decide what to do in terms of treatment?
- In many cases, surgery, radiation, implanted radioactive seeds, or hormone treatment is part of the recommended medical treatment plan. What are the potential side effects of each recommended treatment?
- Have you explored alternative treatments that are not surgical?
- How will the treatment affect your sex life? Are you likely to have urinary problems?
- What are the new treatments that are being offered? Would any of those be appropriate?
- Would a clinical trial be an appropriate choice for you? What are the risks and benefits?

The "Right" Answer

We were committed to pursuing Western treatment options, but we felt there were other options that might also prove beneficial. We decided to take the process in steps to avoid overwhelming ourselves. The first step was to weigh the advantages and risks based on the data we had on from our doctors. Because of our backgrounds in marketing, research, and business, we found ourselves using charts and writing down our evaluations, just as we would in a business situation. This might seem unusual to many people, but with thirty-five years of combined marketing experience between Jim and me, it seemed very natural.

We looked at the options and outcomes and created our own scoring system based on what was important to us. Knowing your grade and stage of cancer will be crucial to determining what treatment options are best for you.

JIM'S PERSONAL EVALUATION OF TREATMENT OPTIONS

Ranked on a 5 Point System* (0–4)
0 no effect, 1 least effective, 2 somewhat effective,
3 effective, 4 most effective

Important Factors	Watchful Waiting	Surgery	Internal Seeds	Cryosurgery	External Radiation	Hormone Therapy / Chemotherapy
Cancer control	0	4	3	2	3	3
Cancer cure (or sense of cure)	0	0–4	3	3	3	2
Urinary dysfunction	0	High risk	Low risk	Low risk	Risk	Low risk
Impotence	N/A	Med. risk	Low risk	Low risk	Risk	High risk (temporary)

*0–4 = Jim and Julia's arbitrary grading scale. Note: You can create your own points and grading system. Note: Internal seeds is a relatively new procedure, but the concept appealed to us because of its precision.

Try filling in the chart below with your own evaluation of the common treatment options and how it relates to your condition.

YOUR OWN EVALUATION OF TREATMENT OPTIONS

Important Factors	Watchful Waiting	Surgery	Internal Seeds	Cryosurgery	External Radiation	Hormone Therapy / Chemo-therapy
Cancer control						
Cancer cure (or sense of cure)						
Urinary dysfunction						
Impotence						

This type of approach helped us understand there were treatments that we probably preferred. However, based on Jim's case, we had to go with the treatment that could be the most successful for him. Surgery was not an option, nor was watchful waiting. Because the disease had spread to his lymph nodes and into the seminal vesicles, radioactive seeds were not going to work. So we decided to pursue a combination of hormone therapy with 3-D radiation and add our own non-Western healing treatments.

The best way to evaluate treatment options is to approach the process with an open mind. Discuss your options freely with your partner or loved ones, and be candid about those details related to potential side effects dend risks. Go into your healing plan with your eyes wide open, and be confident that you have made the best possible choice for yourself based on your individual needs and priorities.

Practically speaking, people with low-grade cancers may do well regardless of the therapy they receive, whereas those with high-grade cancers may not be cured despite the treatment chosen. We learned that many patients with high-grade disease could potentially be undertreated. Paradoxically, people with the most aggressive cases of prostate cancer—like Jim—have received less-aggressive forms of treatment. We believed that Jim should be treated aggressively and with combined treatment modalities, such as hormone therapy and escalated-dose radiation. The doctors agreed that while this aggressive approach may not always be curative, it might improve Jim's chances of survival or prolong his life. There are so many unknown variables with each individual's body and how his disease will respond to treatment, that it really becomes like a probability equation. Each time we learned more about what was available to Jim, we understood there was no clear-cut treatment path. While the doctors had ideas, we were collectively coming up with his course of action.

Many thanks here to Dr. Carroll, Dr. Small, Dr. Phillips, and Dr. Roach, all of whom went out of their way to answer our questions. Because Jim's cancer was outside the prostate, in the lymph nodes, and most likely metastatic, surgery was not an option. The disease was too far-gone. By now we finally believed the cold, hard facts: This was not a tumor we could cut out and dispose of, curing Jim. No, he had to go "through" the cancer and emerge from it healthy and whole. Each cancer cell needed to be eradicated via drugs, radiation, sweating, peeing, crying, or any other way. We had to replace those sick cells with healthy new cells for Jim to be healed and cured. This was going to be hard work, both mentally and physically.

An important part of a successful healing process is to believe that you have the right team of professionals around you. After our visit to UCSF, we knew that it was a place that inspired our confidence and trust, with people we could work with over the long haul. Consequently, Jim and I decided that to work closely with our new partners-in-healing, we would move from Hawaii to San Francisco. Moving a home in the middle of all of this probably sounds crazy, but we felt we had to have some stability during this time. Having our physical possessions available to us was familiar and comfortable. Jim's favorite chair, our pictures, the phone and the alarm clock, our clothes, books, and everything else was like comfort food for the soul. We needed these things in San Francisco to give us a sense of the usual in an extremely unusual time. Despite such a drastic change in lifestyle, the move to San Francisco proved to be a bright spark in our long journey, and we settled down in our new home, ready for the work ahead.

Reaching Beyond the Doctors

Although we had confidence in our doctors, we realized there was a part of us that yearned to think about the disease in a holistic way. Why did Jim get cancer? How could he not only be cured but also be healed? What had we done previously in our lives that we could leverage to help us through this unknown new experience? In other words, we wanted to approach this with a clear goal and focus on creating the best plan and then actively engage in the passionate pursuit of healing Jim.

As we were creating a treatment plan, it became obvious that there was a significant difference between how various philosophies dealt with the disease. The majority of books on Western medicine focus on curing the disease, whereas the alternative and Eastern medical books focused on healing the disease. We learned there is a distinct difference between being healed and being cured. The verb *cure* is defined as "to deal with in a way that eliminated or rectifies," whereas the verb "to heal" is defined as "to make whole and to restore health."

From our perspective, Jim needed to be both healed and cured. Thus we thought about taking advantage of the philosophies and practices of a variety of healing disciplines rather than put all our energy into one form of treatment. Counting on the procedures and drugs from our Western doctors alone did not intuitively seem to be enough to tackle the challenge that life had put before us. We did not want to place all our bets on only one race, one healing option, so we opted for more treatments to complement the Western practices.

Neither Jim nor I had ever done anything like this before, so we talked extensively about the types of actions or activities we were willing to do. We decided we were open to most anything that would create a healing and nurturing environment for Jim. While neither of us had ever participated in alternative medical practices, such as herbs and vitamins, detoxification, or acupuncture, we decided we would actively pursue these treatments to augment the more common and accepted Western medical practices.

If you had surveyed us prior to prostate cancer, we probably would have responded that we would not follow this path. However, as we read more and more, it seemed obvious that there were significant data that supported diet modification, participation in support groups, and alternative medical treatments. Included here are a few of the "facts" we uncovered during our readings, but I would offer the caveat that there are an overwhelming amount of opinions out there, and, ultimately, you have to go with what works for you and what you believe, from the bottom of your heart, will be the best treatment for you. You have to do the soul-searching and determine what is right for you. Be active; don't let the treatment just happen to you. Actively engage in it and use it to heal yourself. Let time and the process work toward making you whole.

PART TWO
TAKING ACTION

DATA TO SUPPORT OUR HOPE

Miracles result from our recognition that even the worst news is only a short story; the whole plot is an unfolding mystery. Be humble in your perpetual uncertainty.

—Paul Pearsall

Ultimately, each body is different and each person reacts to the treatment in a variety of ways. However, there is numerous data available regarding the treatment of various types of prostate cancer. The following is an excerpt from a sample study that was in process while Jim was undergoing his treatments. The study was published in 2001 and the outcome was very encouraging to us. Sample studies can be very important if you are participating in a treatment that still may not be accepted as the normal standard protocol in the medical community. The results from this study prompted Jim's doctors to continue his hormone therapy longer than one or two years. The study shows that there are improved survival rates with extended treatment.

If you are going to a research hospital and facility, ask your doctor what studies they are working on that might be relevant for your prognosis. Our radial oncologist, Dr. Mack Roach, was extensively involved in a series of studies about the levels and applications of radiation in the treatment of advanced prostate cancer.

Sample Study Regarding Advanced Cancer Treatment
(Permission for this section granted by Dr. Mack Roach.
This sample study was segmented for men like Jim.)

Purpose: To assess the impact of short-term and long-term androgen suppression on the disease-specific and overall of 2,200 men treated with radiotherapy in one of five prospective randomized trials when stratified by prognostic risk groups.

Methods and materials: Between 1975 and 1992, 2,742 men were treated for clinically localized prostate cancer. Patients were selected for this analysis if they were deemed able to be evaluated and eligible for the trial, and if follow-up information was available.

Patients were placed in four risk groups. Group 1 and 2 Gleason score under 6, group 3 Gleason score of 7, and Group 4 Gleason score of 8–10.

Results: Group three and four patients were noted to have an approximately 20 percent higher survival at eight years with the addition of long-term hormonal therapy. [This was critical to Jim, having a similar stage, grade, and PSA level.]

Conclusions: These observations should be confirmed by prospective randomized trials before they can be considered conclusive. In the meantime, these observations provide rational guidelines for deciding who should receive hormonal therapy, and for how long.

Disease-Specific Survival Rates

Risk Group	Statistics	Radiation Therapy Alone	Radiation With Longterm Hormone Therapy
2	Death/total Sample	84/443	9/114
	5-year survival rate	94%	93%
	8-year survival rate	83%	89%
3	Death/total sample	96/338	16/132
	5-year survival rate	83%	93%
	8-year survival rate	70%	88%
4*	Death/total sample	154/324	25/103
	5-year survival rate	64%	81%
	8-year survival rate	42%	69%

*Jim was in risk group 4.

This type of quantitative testing and data analysis is vital to patients in their decisionmaking on treatment options and survival.

Radiation Therapy—Are You Cured?

Patients whose PSA levels drop to .02 or below are likely cured of their prostate cancer. But how will they know? During and after radiation therapy, normal and cancerous prostate cells that have received a lethal dose of radiation do not die immediately. The cells will only die when they try to divide. Prostate cancer cells grow slowly, so it can take several years for all cancer cells to die. Even patients in whom every cancer cell is in the radiation-therapy field is destined to die may be unfortunate enough to have cancer cells that have spread to the bone or other areas and that were not irradiated and continue to grow.

Studies show that it can take three years for the PSA to reach its lowest point. For those who are not cured, the cancer cells that grow will ultimately reveal themselves by causing the PSA to increase. Most patients who are likely to develop recurrent prostate cancer do so within four to five years after radiation therapy.

In one study of 328 patients who underwent radiation therapy in doses of roughly 7,400 rads, only three developed recurrent disease after more than five years following radiation therapy. In another study, 446 patients were treated with external-beam radiation. The patients with a PSA greater than 2 nanograms per milliliter after five years did poorly between the fifth to tenth year after radiation therapy. These results indicate that men treated with external-beam radiation do not need to attain and maintain a PSA of .02 nanograms per milliliter to have an excellent chance of being cured.

The current three-dimensional conformal radiation technique uses up to eight different beam positions and custom-shaped metal shields to deliver radiation that is tailored to the prostate gland and the surrounding areas most likely involved with cancer. The percentage of patients free of disease at four years was 41 percent for those treated with the older two-dimensional technique, compared with 61 percent treated with the three-dimensional conformal approach. It should be possible to obtain even better long-term results by placing these men on hormonal therapy for three years. External-beam radiation plus hormonal therapy was more effective after five years than radiation therapy alone.

Prostate cancer patients treated with radiation therapy will often have radiation damage within the normal tissues of the rectum and connecting part of the colon. But other diseases, such as colon cancer, can cause this damage, resulting in diarrhea, bleeding, and rectal pain. That is why the appropriate work up for rectal bleeding usually includes a colonoscopy to look for colon polyps or colon cancer. Unfortunately, heavily irritated rectal and colon tissues are fragile and heal poorly. In a study done by Dr. Dan Theodorescu, of the University of Virginia, of 754 patients who received radiation treatments, seven developed a hole linking their bladder and their bowel. This is a serious complication that leads to bladder infections and a variety of other problems.

Now that you have seen a sample of a research study, you should feel free to ask your doctor if there are any studies that you should be made aware of based on your condition. This disease is going to be controlled through the application of research breakthroughs and new treatments and the commitment of researchers and drug companies.

THE HEALING ACTION PLAN

Man is asked to make of himself what he is supposed to become to fulfill his destiny.

—Paul Tillich

Developing a healing action plan may sound way too formal, too structured, too much like work; however, it became our road map for Jim's healing process. Thoughts were transformed into words, which, in turn, were transformed into actions that ultimately led to our achieving our goal. As we placed the pen in our hands, as we typed the first words on our keyboard, we were beginning to inscribe the message on our brain at the same time. Jim was actively engaging his mind and his body. By *actively engaging*, we mean turning thoughts of the mind into real actions of the body. Thoughts can be the impetus, the beginning of what will be manifested in the body. There has been considerable research on the power of positive thinking for cancer patients. It is evidenced often when placebos are administered, or when someone's will stimulates their body to begin healing itself. We were going to define Jim's healing goals and make them real.

We did not know it at the time but have since come to understand the physical process of this approach. The act of writing neurologically engages a body's reticular activating system (RAS), which is in the brain. The RAS separates and filters urgent from nonurgent information. You become more alert to signs you are on the right path, and the RAS will send your mind signals to reinforce this.

To start the process, define your ultimate goal for the healing plan. What will you say to yourself at the end of your experience with prostate cancer? For Jim it was *I am 100 percent healed and cured.* Here are spirited and aggressive but realistic goals for you to consider for your healing plan:

I am 100 percent cancer free.
I am healed and cured.

I am healthy and happy.
My body, mind, and soul have healed and are cured.
My body is healthy and has killed all the cancer.
I no longer have the disease.

YOUR HEALING GOALS

What is your ultimate healing goal?

What are the steps you can take for your mind, body, and soul to achieve this goal?

Can you put these steps into a timeline to create your plan?

Who else is involved in your plan?

On what date will you start implementing your plan?

What outstanding issues do you need to be aware of?

What is the first step you will take?

This goal will start to become a reality when you develop and write down specific actions that you can take towards achieving it. This will become your Healing Action Plan. Written words are powerful, and each step counts. Once you and your partner know where you want to go, you can start moving toward your destination. Keep that in mind even if the outcome is not exactly as you predicted; taking action towards attaining your goal is progress in and of itself. As an individual or a couple, you are preparing your mind to process and remain committed to the plan by referencing and revising your thoughts and actions.

Maybe at this point you are not so sure of all of this. Then start with a simple first step. Write down a single sentence about what you will be doing as part of your Healing Action Plan.

What one goal can I achieve to help myself in the short term?

If this is still hard, connect with a friend, spouse, or partner. Then both of you should try to write a sentence about the ideas you each have for your healing. This can be the start of your plan; if you have continued difficulty, add at least one action item in seven days and make sure you start to implement it as soon as possible. This allows those freshly minted thoughts to be imprinted in your mind and turn into actions.

What can my friend/partner/spouse do to help himself?

If you have not started to write actions you will take, it is time to consider a change of scenery. Go to an environment that you enjoy, such as a park, an outdoor café, a museum, the mall, or any other place you can think of. Bring a blank pad and a pen. Sit down, relax, and take thirty minutes (or whatever feels right for you), just to be quiet. Don't speak with anyone—just listen to yourself, your inner voice. What is it saying to you? Afterwards pick up your pen and write down the first thoughts that come to your mind. Again, this will be the first step in developing your Healing Action Plan. Don't be surprised if your first thoughts are about how you are feeling. This is your first step in uniting body and mind into one powerful healing force. Acknowledging you are afraid, angry, or anxious is a natural part of the healing process. You cannot run away from these emotions; to help yourself heal, it is vital to work through them.

If this option is not working for you, try another approach. Place a pen and paper by your bed. Before you go to sleep, or, ideally, as soon as you get up, write down your thoughts. Do this for seven days in a row, and do not read what you wrote earlier. On day eight, read all of your writings in one sitting. You will see that you will start to have an idea of what type of actions your Healing Action Plan may include.

SEVEN DAYS OF YOUR THOUGHTS

Day 1

Day 2

Day 3

Day 4
Day 5
Day 6
Day 7

Now, with your goals in mind, you can start to create your plan and take your next steps. Here are some of the subjects you might end up with: diet, relaxation, exercise, treatments, drugs, herbs, vitamins, support group, counseling, therapy, church/synagogue/temple/mosque, social outings, trips, family visits, meditation, self-actualization exercises, and doctors visits. This list is just a sampling of ideas; your list might be similar or totally different.

Your Healing Action Plan is yours and yours alone. It is a way for you to feel empowered and energized. For the ultimate effect, you should do this exercise yourself. No one can write up a complete plan for you without your input. Prepare to take this part of your treatment into your own hands and act, go from being a victim of the cancer to being a victor. Writing it down is an important step. It is a signal to your mind, body, and soul that you are committed to this plan and that these are the steps you are taking to get there.

Questions to Answer

For those with prostate cancer, knowing the answers to these questions will prove instrumental in developing a complete Healing Action Plan.

- *Diet*—Do you need to make any dietary changes that your doctor recommended? Have you removed the cancer-causing foods from your house? Have you purchased any books about healthful eating and living? When will you and your wife/partner talk about making changes to your meals, especially if you are having radiation?
- *Herbs/vitamins*—Did the doctor recommend taking any herbs or vitamins? Are you planning to take vitamin E and

selenium? Do you plan to consult a nutritionist? Do you want to consult an herbalist? Have you set aside time in your day to take the vitamins and reinforce your healing process?

- *Rest/relaxation*—How much rest are you getting per night? While your body is undergoing treatment, are you preparing for the extra rest you need? Could you take ten minutes to a half hour before you sleep to relax, read a book, or just sit quietly in your favorite spot?

- *Exercise*—Do you currently exercise regularly? What is your plan during treatment? How do you plan to retain muscle mass if you are going on hormone treatment? How will you keep your bones strong?

- *Treatments*—Who is your primary doctor? What other doctors or resources are critical for your healing process? What type of treatment will you start? How long will the treatments last?

- *Eastern influence and alternative medicine*—Do you have any desire to pursue Eastern treatments, such as acupuncture? What about yoga? Do you plan to participate in any alternative medicical practices, such as herbal treatments or body cleansing?

- *Spirituality/mental*—Do you mediate? Do you read books on spirituality, self-actualization, or philosophy? Would you try biofeedback, *reiki* (a Japanese healing art), stress relief, or counseling? Do you go to church, temple, or other place of worship? Could you make any of these activities part of your weekly healing? Do you pray? Have you ever been in a spiritual group?

- *Support*—Do you plan on attending support groups? Alone? With your spouse or significant other? Are you aware of any support groups at your hospital, in your community, or at your place of worship?

- *Weight*—Do you have a few extra pounds you might want to shed? How many pounds, and how fast? (Be realistic, so you don't disappoint yourself—some treatment drugs actually can cause weight gain.)

Notes From Jim's Healing Action Plan

Included here are initial notes that helped us form Jim's Healing Action Plan:

TREATMENT NOTES

Date of first treatment	Description of initial medication or procedure LHRH agonist (analog) + Casodex—complete hormone deprivation *Notes:* Dr. Chinn administered–need to schedule appt. for PSA test in 1 month March 17 Dr. Clayton Chung visit set w/time for additional tests set Description of subsequent medication or procedure Chinese herbal treatment—based on Chinese herbalist Vitamin E Selenium 1,000 mg vitamin C extra/day
Date of change or additional treatment	*Notes:* Herbalist provided Jim with one month supply of herbs Three kinds of important herbs: 1. Herbs that support immune system 2. Herbs that promote health of liver 3. Herbs that help immune system eliminate toxins Description of any further medication or procedure Examination by Drs. Phillips, Carroll, Small UCSF—Discussion of aggressive 3-D radiation treatment to be done at UCSF . . . Radiation levels to exceed accepted norms
Date of any change in treatment	*Notes:* Additional treatment of radiation to be added after 4 months of Casodex & LHRH–will include 8 weeks or more of radiation–daily–"cure" is the goal—radiation + 1–2 years hormone therapy . . . Herbs/vitamins to stop them

<table>
<tr><td></td><td>Description of any further medication or procedure

LHRH (analog) shot 1 mo. dose
PSA test results—April 7—1.1—Wow!</td></tr>
<tr><td>Date of any change in treatment</td><td>*Notes:*
Hemoglobin blood count less
Short-term disability note signed effective May 1
Dr. Chun agrees w/radiation therapy exploration

Based on reading—added:
Olive oil diet replaces all oils and fats in our
Saw-palmetto, soy isoflavines (genestein)–3x1
Located an acupuncturist and will begin treatment in May</td></tr>
<tr><td>Date of any change in treatment</td><td>*Notes:*
Continuation of all other treatments—Jim sweats some and his weight is in check. Mentally A+ with lots going on inside</td></tr>
</table>

From the time Jim received his first treatment (the Lupron shot and Casodex), the goal was to continue with them for another three months and hope the tumor would shrink before the radiation treatment started. Fortunately, the tumor did shrink, and Jim's PSA dropped significantly from over 39 to below 1.1. This was a good sign, because it indicated that at least part of the cancer depended on testosterone to grow. The effect of the shrinking tumor would make it easier to focus the radiation on the remaining cancerous area. We were on our way to destroying the prostate cancer cells. Our goal: to kill each devious, life-threatening cancer cell.

Now, after what had seemed like years, we initiated the beginning of Jim's Healing Action Plan. We finally had an initial phase of the plan, because we had determined the treatment type, the doctors, and the timing. Patience is required—you may want to act immediately, but first you need to determine who is on your healing team and the vision you have for your personal healing plan before you initiate meaningful action. Our next step was to decide on alternative and Eastern healing techniques that would make our traditional Western medicine treatment plan more holistic, more encompassing of body, mind, and soul.

To give an idea of how we organized and planned our Healing Action Plan, we included daily, weekly, and monthly activities. The plan included physical, mental, and emotional activities. This type of plan enabled Jim to feel that he was actively participating in the healing process. As his critical caregiver and main supporter, it was vitally important to me as well. It made us active participants, as opposed to passive receivers of doctor's instructions, drugs, and treatments.

To put it in perspective, there are many activities you can include in a long-term healing process. Here are some of the items we included:

DAILY	**WEEKLY**	**MONTHLY**
Exercise/ running	Support group	Attend prostate-cancer conferences
Sauna	Doctors' visits	
Herbs and vitamins	Acupuncture	Medical tests
Sleep—eight hours, minimum	Church	Plan day and vacation trips
Radiation (for four months)	Weight training	Lunch w/ prostate-cancer survivors
Pray/visualize/ meditate	Flowers— beautiful, living	
Daily drugs & hormone therapy	Dinner out with family/friends	

Executing Your Healing Action Plan

By taking the time to consider your options and asking yourself some exceedingly difficult questions, you will learn more about what is important in your life. Be prepared to discover many things about yourself, the ones you love, and the beautiful gift of life. This is a gift we all have been fortunate enough to receive, and even though you've been delivered this challenge, try to cherish life.

- What is the healing and treatment plan you are going to pursue?
- Do I need to take off work?
- How long will the treatment take?
- Is it covered by insurance? If not, how will I fund the treatments?
- How do I plan to manage my social life during the treatment?
- Do I have any obstacles I need to remove to accomplish my healing goal?
- Have I written my plan down?
- Am I updating the plan with new information?
- Am I having any side effects that I should make the doctor aware of?
- What am I going to do to make sure I am staying on my plan?
- Will I be weighing myself?
- If daily treatments are required, how do I plan to stick to them?
- Am I committed to listening to my body and checking physical signs, such as my urine and stool, daily for abnormalities?
- Am I committed to reporting side effects in a timely matter? Will I note and share my observations with my doctor? If I have any changes in my plan, will I be sure to document them?
- Am I making sure to monitor my attitude? Am I compassionate to myself when I can't be positive?
- Have I started to write down my plan or track it in another way?

After all that you have read in this book and the questions you've answered above, you are well on your way to making a personalized Healing Action Plan. It takes time and energy to start your plan, but as you begin to implement it, you will see the actions of your thoughts and words manifesting themselves. This is rewarding and can serve as your road map to complete the Circle of Healing.

We found as we implemented Jim's plan that we added things over time and that taking it step-by-step was the best way to achieve our healing goal. We wanted to make sure we were always on the road, looking up the mountain instead of sliding down the slippery slope of self-pity, inactivity, and despair. Jim was exhausted and having "long blinks"—falling asleep while sitting up—he tried to engage in life and the magnitude of the situation seemed insurmountable, but the initiative of developing a healing plan and goal helped us turn what was physically and emotionally exhausting into a replenshing reservoir of life. We used the following chart to prepare for our doctor's visits during our treatment plan. We discussed the answers to these questions with our doctor during each visit, especially if there had been a noticeable change from our previous visit. This was a nifty way to monitor Jim's body and provide the doctor with meaningful information he needed to know.

Circle the number in the column that best describes your situation.	Not at all	Less than 1 time in 5	Less than half the time	About half the time	More than half the time	Almost always
1. Over the past month, how often have you had the sensation that your bladder is not completely empty after you finish urinating?	0	1	2	3	4	5
2. Over the past month, how often have you had to urinate again in less than 2 hours since the last time?	0	1	2	3	4	5

Circle the number in the column that best describes your situation.	Not at all	Less than 1 time in 5	Less than half the time	About half the time	More than half the time	Almost always
3. Over the past month, how often have you you stopped and started again several times when urinating?	0	1	2	3	4	5
4. Over the past month, how often have you found it difficult to postpone urination?	0	1	2	3	4	5
5. Over the past month, how often have you had a weak urinary stream?	0	1	2	3	4	5
6. Over the past month, how often have you had to push or strain to begin urination?	0	1	2	3	4	5

	None	1 time	2 times	3 times	4 times	5 times
7. Over the past month, how many times did you most typically get up to urinate from the time you went to bed at night to the time you got up in the morning?	0	1	2	3	4	5

	Extremely satisfied	Very satisfied	satisfied	Neutral	Slightly dissatisfied	dissatisfied
8. If you were to spend the rest of your life with your urinary condition the way it is now, how would you feel about it?	0	1	2	3	4	5

Total Score (sum of all numbers circled):

Modified from a form provided by UCSF Urology Dept., 2002

Stay Current

Sometimes it is hard to stay on top of everything going on in the world, but knowledge of cancer and its treatment is important. This can mean the difference between life and death, the difference between a full recovery and a partial recovery. To help us stay current, we employed several techniques that allow information to come to us via subscription and updates. Jim has also stayed active in a high-level, future-oriented prostate-cancer advocate group hosted by UCSF.

Part of the advantage of getting newsletters and updates is they are subtle reminders that you are a person who has or who had cancer, and that you are very fortunate to be on this earth at this moment. There is highly significant research going on right now for prostate cancer, and the knowledge derived from clinical trials initiated years ago is just starting to be presented at doctors' panels, ultimately to reach patients.

The one publication that both Jim and I read cover to cover is the *Prostate Forum Newsletter,* published by Dr. Charles Myers of Charlottesville, Virginia. It is available via e-mail at www.prostateforum.com. Believe it or not, during our three-year journey, this doctor actually found out he had prostate cancer and published his selection of treatment options. One of the things we noticed was that he was quite specific about making sure he treated all potential sources of testosterone generation in his body. This, too, was a strategy we had employed in Jim's treatment. Adding Proscar to Lupron, Casodex, and Fosomax seemed unnecessary three years ago, but two years later a knowledgeable doctor was taking the same drugs to treat his cancer.

The newsletter covers many aspects of prostate cancer and usually discusses one topic and three to four subjects relating to the topic. It only takes thirty to forty-five minutes to read, but it is packed with information and provides reminders of current treatments.

Often the newsletter becomes the starting point for a conversation between Jim and I about his treatment. It is a way for us to initiate discussion about what is on his mind, without him feeling he is dwelling on the cancer. Of course, there are other ways to stimulate conversation about cancer and feelings, but this is one positive and educational approach.

As mentioned earlier, support groups are critical. Even after Jim had been involved in one for more than a year he knew he needed more. We contacted UCSF to find out whether more were available and whether it offered additional types of education and prostate-cancer support groups. It turned out that we were pretty up-to-date on current treatments because of the newsletters and journals we read. However, the support groups added the human element to the healing process. Fortunately, UCSF has a quarterly meeting, Prostate Advocates, to discuss future treatments of prostate cancer, as well as other advancements in knowledge about prostate cancer. Jim goes to these quarterly meetings, which are well attended and include lectures on prostate cancer by some of the best minds in the world. A plus is that the meeting is only a thirty-minute drive from home.

Various meetings like these take place in different cities all around the United States and include a variety of guest speakers from visiting hospitals in addition to many men from the local community. Seek these types of events in your area. They are inspiring, educational, and bonding. They can help you get through the ongoing process and keep a smile on your face by being able to laugh, commiserate, and accept what is happening. Share and bond with compatriots, those people with prostate cancer, their spouses, and their doctors. This can all be a part of the healing process and your support system.

Working to Live Versus Living to Work

One of the major changes we made in our lives was our approach to work. Prior to Jim's diagnosis, we both spent an enormous amount of time working. When we found out that Jim had cancer, we were thrown into a disorienting dilemma. We both had so much of our identity wrapped up in who we were at work rather than who we were as individuals. We had been nicely rewarded with the luxurious trappings of an executive life; however, once we found out about the cancer work no longer seemed as important. Unless you are actually living through a similar situation, this might be difficult to understand, but we found it was possible to change suddenly and dramatically when we realized how short life can be.

Jim had held senior management positions for the last fifteen years. He had been the president of some companies and an executive vice president of others. The titles themselves were really not as relevant as the amount of work and responsibility that came with them. Company performance, profitability, the well-being of the company's associates—Jim was giving too much energy to his work. His body was totally depleted. He had no more to give. In fact, this giving had brought him to the point where a disease was killing him. He had to take a step back and start to replenish his energy, his body, and his mind. He needed to do things now that would put energy back into the "Jim battery."

Jim approached his employer, LVMH (Louis Vuitton Moet Hennessey/DFS), to allow him to go on disability while he was getting treated. The company was absolutely fantastic about understanding why he had to do this and allowed us the full flexibility we needed. For the first year of treatment, his company provided Jim with some disability. In subsequent years we handled the payments ourselves by establishing our own marketing services company, Real eMarketing. This gave Jim and me the flexibility we needed to make his treatments our number-one priority. It was ideal for us. Had the cancer not have caused us to dramatically rethink what we were doing, we probably would have stayed on the same grueling work schedule for the next ten or twenty years. Who knows what other health problems this may have caused?

Jim and I worked together, traveled together, and lived together, a magnificent way to go through his healing and experience. As an added benefit, this gave us a chance to see a whole different side of business and work. We became much more independent and further developed skills such as being able to use computer programs and information technology comfortably, learning tricks about airline traveling, and appreciating all the aspects of what it takes to run a company.

Suddenly, enjoying every moment of our lives together became our top priority. Whether those moments are spent just talking, running, or being with family and friends, they are what really matter. For Jim, the change was almost immediate; for me, it has taken longer, for several reasons. I was not the one whose life was in danger. I was Jim's main support, and assumed a host of responsibilities because of this new role. I had to be right in the thick of all the real-life noise out there. While trying to shield Jim from those annoyances, I was caught up with the overwhelming details of day-to-day life.

Even today, Jim grounds me by reminding me of what is really important in life rather than what seems to be important in the moment. Undoubtedly, the fact is that he was the one who lived through cancer, and the impact of this experience was different for each of us. His experience was so much more intense and disrupted internally by the disease. As head caregiver, info researcher, patient advocate, and more, there is a fair amount of emotional trauma that comes with this responsibility. I often found myself emotionally drained, very worried, and having trouble sleeping. This was not a normal state for me. I was so wound up inside. Looking back, it was all part of the experience of having prostate cancer in my life. The good news is, I was able to emerge from it a stronger, more complete person.

When trying to cope with cancer, you must do whatever you can to remove stress and improve work and family situation. People may not be able to change their work arrangement in an ideal situation, but every option to make improvements needs to be explored. Cancer patients cannot afford to be overcome with stress, as this interferes with healing and curing. As a preventative measure, it is important to make sure that your company offers both short- and long-term disability insurance and to always opt-in for that coverage if you are offered that option. Healing takes support.

Summary of Our Healing Action Plan

One important step we took was to summarize the healing plan we had been carrying out the last three years. It was a great way for us to capture on paper how far we had come. It is easier to see now, compared with when we started out, how a clear goal becomes a beacon for the journey. These are the highlights of the three years of our healing plan, summarized in a simple chart:

OUR GOAL: TO HEAL AND CURE JIM

Prostate-cancer cells are capable of committing suicide. This process of self-destruction can be triggered by Jim taking the following actions:

<table>
<tr>
<td>Understanding cancer-cell destruction</td>
<td>

- When testosterone is removed following medical advice with hormone therapy.
- When we treat prostate cancer with radiation.
- When cancer chemotherapy drugs are taken.
- When Genistein is administered at high levels.
- *Important fact:* If you're still in remission five years after external-beam radiation therapy, odds are you've been cured.
- In July Jim begins radiation therapy and finishes in late September due to increased dosage level.

</td>
</tr>
<tr>
<td>Traditional treatment</td>
<td>

- In a follow up conversation with Dr. Roach, we ask him to explore Jim's history again and if he can do anything else. The doctor comes back and we aggressively pursue Jim's fight with more radiation. The final level of radiation is 8200 rads.
- Radiation therapy included 3-D conformal radiation to the prostate gland, seminal vesicles, and pelvic lymph nodes.

</td>
</tr>
<tr>
<td>Radiation therapy</td>
<td>

- Months after radiation therapy, patients can develop a PSA that peaks and then drops to a low level consistent with remission, a phenomenon called the PSA bump. Jim did not, and his PSA remains below .02 (undetectable).
- Jim begins to have rectal bleeding and we have to rule out colon cancer.
- Slight bleeding continues, but there are no other side effects at this time.
- Jim had been diagnosed with prostate cancer in January. He had three

</td>
</tr>
</table>

<table>
<tr><td valign="top">Complementary treatments = TOTAL healing & treatment</td><td>

years with androgen-withdrawal, using Lupron, Casodex, and Proscar. He began to lose his body hair everywhere but his head within six months.

- Fosomax was added and used to prevent osteoporosis.
- Twice-weekly acupuncture visits, then reduced to weekly visits after two years.
- Aggressive use of herbs and vitamins starting, modified three times since initial treatment, then during radiation, after radiation, and after removal from all the hormone therapy and other drugs.
- Jim begins weight training for the first time in June and still continues a five times-a-week routine now. Jim exercises every day by running about three to four miles (he already was exercising prior to finding out about the cancer).
- Over three years after diagnosis, his PSA remains less than .02 ng/ml. After radiation therapy, nearly all relapses occur during the first five years. He now has less than two years until he will be in the clear.
- Jim is removed from all prostate-cancer drugs after three years, with the exception of Proscar. He remains on Fosomax.
- Jim still continues with daily exercise, herbs and vitamins, diet consciousness, and prayer.
- Great news five months after treatment: Jim's PSA is .05, and his testosterone level is above 600.
- Weekly church, musical, entertainment, or spiritual event; bimonthly acupuncture or massage.
- Monthly newsletter reading.
- Quarterly, he gets his PSA tested and attends support group meetings.
- Becomes active in UCSF Prostate Advocates Group.

</td></tr>
</table>

- Two years later, MRI done, no detectable metastic cancer, seminal vesicles and prostate clear PSA .18
- Jim has less than one year until his doctor will give him additional confidence that the cancer is not an issue.

COMMITTING MIND, BODY, AND SOUL

Your desire is your prayer. Picture the fulfillment of your desire now and feel its reality and you will experience the joy of the answered prayer.

—Dr. Joseph Murphy

With your thoughts, you have tremendous control over what happens to your body and how the prostate cancer impacts your spirit. Another great benefit of positive thinking is that it is free. Your thoughts are free, and you can have total individual control of how you choose to react and process the information you are receiving and creating within your mind.

While getting settled into a completely new routine—one of doctors, acupuncturists, herb stores, pharmacies, and the like—you are suddenly exposed to a whole different world, a world of invasive dis-ease, negative thought, and stress that keeps making people who are sick get sicker. Quite frankly, it is important when in the hospital, at the doctor's office, and in treatment rooms to think positive thoughts. It requires adjusting your mind to think of those places as spaces in the world where you go to be cured and healed, not because you are sick. Ironically, going there is a part of the route to not having to go there. It is a step on the path to healing, like forging a path up a mountain. Each action and deed along the way moves you further and further up the mountain. You can leave behind where you were and exist in a new place that is better and healthier. Each step planted to reach the summit of the mountain without fear of looking back or fear of what is to come is true progress.

In terms of attaining riches in life, there is an old expression about paying yourself first. The concept speaks to when you earn money, paying yourself first by saving a percentage of your proceeds right off the top. The ideal outcome is that then you will live a life without being in need of as much money as you would have needed had you not been saving. For people who are fighting cancer the saying should be modified to, "Take care of yourself first—"

not in a selfish way, but in a way whereby priorities are in the right order. Given that prostate cancer can kill you, if you let it grow and flourish, you may die. For Jim to emerge from prostate cancer, we realized that his energy should be focused on healing and curing. The most important thing you can do is to prepare for the fight, clearly believing that "my body and mind can fight this, will beat this." It is a fight, a struggle, but you have to take it head on, go right through it, and come out the other side. There are no shortcuts. Cancer is a ruthless and vile enemy of your body. It turns a body against itself in the cruelest form of abuse. Cell by cell, it kills happy, healthy cells and replaces them with destructive, malignant cells.

The greater the magnitude of the disease, the greater the energy needed to fight it, to overcome it. Think about the laws of physics: For every action in the universe, there is an equal and opposite reaction. If the cancer is strong and deadly, the reaction to it should be that, you must fight back more strongly to overcome it. To bring the body back to a balanced and healthy state, one must overcompensate with healthy actions, thoughts, and deeds to get back to an equilibrium.

Life is precious and yet often we get caught up in the day-to-day and forget to appreciate—to say thanks and be grateful for our lives. If you do not believe in God and praying is not for you that is fine. At least take time to appreciate the fact that you are alive and a part of this amazing universe, with all its wonder and glory.

Meditation and Prayer

Certainly one outcome of prostate cancer is the realization that you cannot deal with it entirely alone. One way we coped with illness was by going to church. We are blessed to live within four blocks of Grace Cathedral, a beautiful Gothic church situated at the top of Nob Hill in San Francisco. The grandness and beauty of the cathedral provided us with a sense of the spiritual power and energy of the universe. The sheer size and proportion of the space let us know that we are a small part of an existence and a reality that is much more significant than ours. The feeling of peace and warmth emanating from the sun shining through the stained-glass windows soothes the soul, the grandeur of the Gothic columns provides a sense of power and might beyond what is visible to the naked eye, and the quietness and peace provide serenity for calming the body.

We try to attend the 7:30 A.M. service on most Sundays while in San Francisco. The first service of the morning seems quiet and reserved (maybe because we are all still partially waking up) and is attended only by an intimate group of around twenty-five other parishioners and out-of-town visitors. This is hard to imagine, because the church has the capacity to hold over two thousand attendees.

When we are out of town, we try on occasion to locate a local church, regardless of the denomination. If we don't do that, we try to engage in some other type of social and spiritual activity— seminars, blessings, or appreciative ceremonies like parades. The symbolism of these activities is helpful to one's spirit and serves as a powerful reinforcement of the wonder and appreciation of life.

The time we spend in church is one in which we acknowledge there is so much more to healing Jim than just what we can control. We have needed God to help us cope and accept what was happening in dealing with cancer. Often the sermons seem to have points of reference to the sick and the struggle for life. It is a way for us to understand we can live with dignity with the disease, to realize that self-love and forgiveness are important to being a fulfilled person. We have learned to be true to ourselves and not judge or be critical of others. Unconditional acceptance of what is, not meaning to roll over and say, "Oh, woe is me!" but to graciously interact with others and love them, to be true to yourself and others, and to pray to God to be healed and cured. While we are in church, we pray for others in our family, our friends, and the many people in the world in need.

We realize that some form of spiritual practice each day, whether it is prayer or meditation, is a wonderful habit to add to one's life. This daily routine can give you tremendous spiritual peace even though you are in emotional and physical turmoil.

Elizabeth Kubler-Ross said, "Learn to get in touch with the silence within yourself and know that everything in this life has a purpose." Depending on your personality, you can work consciously on a daily basis to meditate, create, develop and stay focused on positive thoughts. Whether or not you are a religious person, the act of praying, meditating, or saying positive affirmations is like calling to your body, "Listen! This is important!" It helps you remove all the clutter from your life for at least a few minutes and allows your body the time to hear a positive message being sent from your mind. Your mind can, to some extent, exercise control and discipline over your body. Praying or meditating—quietly saying a short statement like, "I want my body to be healed and cured"—is a significant act for those seeking to heal. This is a simple and understandable message that, when sent without noise of interruption, is pure and powerful.

The power of positive thinking and prayer of others had a positive impact on Jim's healing process. Jim had hundreds of family members, friends, coworkers, and the church praying for him. All those moments our friends and family gave to Jim were appreciated beyond words. Whether directly or indirectly, this helped Jim to heal and be cured. To all those who prayed and sent well wishes, positive thoughts, and prayers, they worked, and we are eternally grateful.

Affirmations and Self-Actualization

An alternative to praying or meditating is practicing positive affirmations. Jerry Frankhauser said, "Affirmations are like prescriptions for certain aspects of yourself you want to change." They are statements that you can make to yourself privately or out loud. Try one of the affirmations below or create your own. Finding one that you wholeheartedly believe in is critical to maximizing the power of affirmations.

POSITIVE AFFIRMATIONS

Thank you for healing and curing me.

Thank you for all the blessings in my life.

Thank you for giving me the strength to heal and cure.

Thank you for the love of my life.

Thank you for giving me the strength to be the best I can be to heal and cure.

Write down one of your own or repeat one from above.

Fill your heart and your mind with thoughts like this when you are ill. Don't let your mind go into a negative spiral from all the issues. Be positive, be happy, and create happy, healthy cells. Think about your body as a large manufacturer of cells. Every day it makes millions of cells, and you want each of them to be happy and healthy; you want to fill your body with only healthy cells as the cancerous cells die off.

Another technique for positive thinking is the concept of self-actualization. It might sound self-indulgent or only for people that are into New Age thinking, but it is not. The Eastern religion of Zen deals with being with oneself and the universe, manifesting thoughts into reality, and achieving inner peace. In Mazlow's *Heirarchy of Needs,* the last level, or highest need, is self-actualization—making yourself the best you can be, taking control of your life, and turning your dreams or goals into reality. Affirmations are useful to the process of self-actualization.

One of Jim's healing action items was his daily round of self-actualization exercises. This was a great way for him to maintain a positive attitude in the face of cancer and, at the same time, actively care for his mind and body. When Jim and I are running together, we often repeat the following affirmations like an army drill:

> *Love life.*
> *Love God.*
> *Heal Jim.*
> *Cure Jim.*

With each step on our left foot, "Love," on our right foot, "life," left, "Love," right, "God," left, "Heal," right, "Jim," cure, "Jim," and repeat. It makes it fun, and takes my mind off my shortness of breath! At the end of our runs, I am thankful for being able to run another day with Jim, and each step marks another step on our path to self-actualization. After starting on this positive note, we go on our way into the day.

Below are a few affirmations to aid your own self-actualization. Make them to yourself throughout the day, at work, in a meeting that is a waste of time, in a checkout line, while exercising, in the shower, or anywhere else. Be in the moment and focus on the thought. Say these words out loud or to yourself. Believing in this process has been profoundly energizing to us.

SELF-ACTUALIZATION STATEMENTS

Thank you for healing me.

Thank you for curing me.

Thank you for making me healthy and strong.

Thank you for making me sexually vibrant.

Release all my past anger.

Release all the cancer cells from my body.

Make happy, healthy cells.

Love life, love God, and cure me.

Treat me with the divine energy of the universe.

Forgive me; heal me.

Give me the energy to heal others and myself.

Make me whole, cure me, and heal me.

These actualization statements can be said by a loved one on behalf of another as well. Mental self-affirmations are critical. Your mind gives instructions to your body. Try to stop letting the mind be the victim of the body. Any of these affirmations can work, or try constructing one for yourself.

SELF-AFFIRMATIONS

Write your affirmation here:

____

Now say it aloud.

Now silently.

Now aloud.

Now silently.

Now aloud.

By placing your mind in action, you can begin to see yourself as you describe your personal Circle of Healing. The path of creating a successful healing process is not always direct, but having a great mental attitude can help you make it through the challenge.

Visualization

Another important technique that is part of the power of positive thinking is visualization. The power of visualization has been used to heal a variety of physical conditions. It clears the mind of distractions and allows an individual to focus on aligning his or her body, mind, and soul. The best-seller *Getting Well Again* by Carl Simonton and Stephanie Simonton documented that in early 1971 a group of cancer patients survived because they had the will to live and participated in visualization. Jean Achtenberg joined with the Simontons to develop a criterion for effective imagery for healing. Since their work was done almost thirty years ago, it is amazing how focused they were on the power of the mind, body, and soul working together.

Here are examples of the types of visualizations they encouraged their patients to see in their minds. Go ahead and picture these images in your mind.

VISUALIZATIONS

See cancer cells as weak and confused, falling apart.

View your treatment as a strong and powerful warrior.

Healthy cells repair themselves easily; if they are damaged by the treatment, they heal themselves easily.

A massive army of all types of white blood cells is overwhelming the cancer cells.

White blood cells want to attack and kill the cancer cells.

Dead cancer cells are leaving your body in every way, through every pore; they are flushed out, cried out, breathed out, and sweated out.

See yourself as healthy and cancer free.

See yourself realizing your goals and fulfilling your legacy.

During Jim's daily routine of radiation treatments, he actively visualized the cancer leaving his body, through his sweat, pee, tears, bowel movements, and breath. We often made references to his purging of all those dead cancer cells and having them replaced with happy, healthy cells. This was a powerful mental image Jim could see in his mind. His mind worked together with his body to make this a reality.

Having the right mental attitude is crucial, and there are many personal ways to get there. Determine a plan that is right for you as an individual and commit your mind and soul to the plan. It is vital that you align and balance your body, mind, and soul on the effort of healing. It requires the entire essence of your being to be actively engaged in the healing process.

Now you have a few ideas concerning how to place positive thoughts in your mind. There is not a lot of research on this; it is truly a matter of having faith and trust in existence and reality outside of your control.

Negative Versus Positive Thoughts

Jim and I were not optimistic one hundred percent of the time throughout our battle with cancer, but we learned that we had to see the possibility of hope and act on it. We redirected negative thoughts into alternative thoughts for coping and healing. Here are some examples of the thoughts Jim had and how he was able to positively interpret them.

NEGATIVE THOUGHTS	POSITIVE THOUGHTS
1. I'm hopeless and there is nothing I can do.	1. Each person is different, and my initial response to treatment is positive.
2. It's my fault—I'm going to die and leave my family without a father.	2. I don't know that I am going to die. My doctors believe there is a chance for me.
3. The doctor isn't telling me everything.	3. The doctor is telling me what he knows at this time, but he cannot guarantee results.
4. If someone rejects me, I must be worthless.	4. No matter who rejects me, I'm still a desirable and valuable person.

You may be the type of person who often has negative thoughts, but that doesn't mean you shouldn't feel the way you feel. It only means you have an opportunity to ask yourself why you feel that way. Getting in touch with your emotional health puts you in a place where you can reflect on who you are and why you are that way. It is only natural. Deciphering your thoughts and accepting them is a healthy and vital part of the healing process.

If you fail to understand why you are thinking and feeling negative thoughts, you are apt to behave in ways that may hurt yourself and others. You are not as likely to end up with the healing outcome you want. Take the time to evaluate your negative thoughts. Is the thought negative because you are angry at the cancer? Do you hate it? Do you feel betrayed by your body? Are you ashamed that you are now weak? Do you have fear that you will lose your masculinity? These types of negative thoughts are natural. The issue is how you process them in your mind.

Take time to acknowledge that you have the right to feel that way, but rather than acting from fear and anger with negative energy, you need to let go of those thoughts and consciously replace them with positive ones. Each time you do this, you will start to train your mind to stay focused on the present and to produce positive thoughts that will ultimately assist in your overall well-being. Try filling in the chart below with your own thoughts.

NEGATIVE THOUGHTS	POSITIVE THOUGHTS
1.	1.
2.	2.
3.	3.

Your body, mind, and soul are united and, as such, need to go through this disease unified and positive. Try one of the powerful techniques provided earlier, or create your own. Finding a statement you really believe in is the most important part of the exercise.

ACUPUNCTURE

Trust that still, small voice that says, "This might work, and I'll try it."

—Diane Mariechild

In our quest for alternative treatments to supplement the Western treatments that Jim was receiving, we were intrigued with acupuncture. Living in San Francisco among so much Chinese-influenced culture made us more open and excited about the potential of this ancient Asian healing art, whose principles are based on traditions from more than 5,000 years ago.

Our first encounter with acupuncture was quite intense. The session started with a series of questions about Jim's past. Many questions were difficult to answer—questions about past relationships; what makes one happy or sad; past illnesses; family history; personal frustrations, and personal desires and passions.

I stayed with Jim for the entire time, and I saw him go through what I can only describe as a metamorphosis, after the interview, called traditional diagnosis. The room was very hot, and Jim stripped down and lay under blankets. Utterly exhausted, he quickly dozed after the earlier questioning. This clearly is a part of allowing past emotions to become uncorked. Unknown sources of pain, many past hurts—we all have them, and, like seeds of destruction planted deep in our soul, they need to be removed, flushed out forever, or we risk that they will grow at some other time into disease. As Jim says, they are tiny grains of rice that get stored into a box within yourself. Eventually the box becomes stuffed and bursts open. Prostate cancer was the manifestation of Jim's rice box bursting.

After the round of questions plus the brief nap, the acupuncturist came in and set a full set of needles down. I sat up, fully alert. I asked to pick one up. It seemed improbable to me that this tiny little needle, smaller than the ones I use for sewing, could do much of anything. But after reading about acupuncture, the idea that a body has energy flows that will be aided by these tiny needles, made practical sense to me.

What happened next was utterly amazing. With a sense of calm and authority, Peggy began to touch Jim at certain parts of his body. At his wrists, she felt his pulse points. She said he had a lot of blockages, but that this was normal, especially with all he had going on in his body. Next she informed us the first part of his rebalancing could be as short as an hour or as long as three or four, depending on how he responded. This was new for Jim and me, but we calmly accepted it as a part of the process. I sat by and watched as Peggy, a master acupuncturist with more than twenty years of experience, began to work on Jim's body.

With precision, she started placing pins all over his body. On occasion he would utter a slight ow, but, in general, it was totally painless. As he lay on his stomach, she placed alot of needles into critical energy spots on his back.

What was interesting, was what was happening around the needles. In some places they fell out on their own within a minute, just as she had said. In other cases, there were small red patches around the needles; it looked as though there were little raspberries on Jim's back. In one area, which we learned later was the heart protector, the patch was as big and as red as an oversize strawberry. Not only was it large, but it was very red, as if blood was gathering there, the needle trying to help his body excise the poison as soon as possible. It was fascinating to see this.

Jim was calm and relaxed, a great patient who accepted the treatment and did not rush the process. All the emotional stress and the initiation of his hormone shots and pills had so worn him out that he was able to doze off. I sat there and watched for about the first forty-five minutes as the needles started to be "released"—and with them, Jim's blockages from years earlier. As the next hour passed, I sat on a couch and started to rest. Everything was taking a toll on me as well; I, too, was tired and had such sadness in my heart. Truly, my heart was aching. I'd been sad before, but never had I felt the sensation of my heart aching with pain.

By now almost two hours had passed, and there were only a few needles remaining. During this time Peggy and her assistant were checking on us to make sure we were comfortable.

Over three-and-a half hours passed before the needle that was surrounded by the "strawberry" (which had developed in under five minutes) fell out and all signs of the redness were gone. Jim was through his first major step in rebalancing his *qi*, his life-energy force.

The way he describes it, he felt light—not a magical "I'm cured," but lighter and relieved. Maybe the needles had acted as conduits for the release of years of pent-up disease that had led him to such illness.

With so much at stake, we were absolutely dedicated to placing as many positives in his healing account as possible. To us, acupuncture was just one more ingredient in the entire healing process. During radiation and the intensive "attack the cancer" phase, Jim went to acupuncture three times a week. He looked forward to the time, the peace and the release for his body. It was one of those special times he had when he sent loud-and-clear signals to his body, mind, and spirit, "I love you and want you to be well." As Jim's body started to get stronger and adjust to the drugs, after radiation he went once a week for the next year and a half. Now he goes to acupuncture once every two weeks. There is no doubt that after a session he comes home relaxed—released.

This channel of non-Western therapy helped Jim slow down, to take time to contemplate all that was going on around and in him. It was one more way to reinforce in his mind, body, and spirit that healing was most important. His actions were helping his mind prepare his character for being a healthy, well-balanced human being.

The Principles of Acupuncture

The vast difference between traditional Western medical practices and Eastern methods is traditional Chinese medicine does not treat symptoms. According to Chinese teachings, whatever happens naturally outside us also happens within us. In the Chinese system of acupuncture healing, we are an extension of cosmic energy. In Western medicine, doctors specialize in particular body parts that are not well. In this Eastern system of medicine, a person is viewed not as parts but as one entire being. Any part of us that is not functioning correctly must affect the whole. Additionally, the part affected is not necessarily the cause; it may only be the surface symptom. The disease is being caused internally by a variety of conditions, such as worry, fear, grief, hostility, anger, hatred, and jealousy, or external causes, like wind, heat, dryness, cold, humidity, chemical causes or mechanical causes of disease. The primary emphasis of the Chinese system of medicine is the ability to diagnose the root cause of the disease.

In acupuncture it is believed that in our body we have ten officials. The ten officials are heart, small intestines, bladder, kidney, gall bladder, liver, lungs, colon, stomach and spleen. In addition, it is thought that the body has two functions: Circulation-Sex and Three Heater. Circulation-Sex governs all internal and external sexual secretions; it's also referred to as the pericardium-Heart Protector. The energy is physical, mental, and spiritual. The function has control over love, joy, laughter, and well-being. The Three-Heater function is named as such because the body is divided into three areas, termed *jiaos*. Each person has an upper, middle, and lower *jiao*, which keep the organs at the right temperature to function normally. The temperatures of each should be identical so that there is complete balance in your body. If they aren't, there will be imbalance and your body will ultimately develop some form of disease.

If the organs and the functions are working in balance and harmony as nature ordains, it is impossible to be sick in body, mind, or spirit. Every disease in the world is caused by one or more of the ten officials not functioning correctly. As an official starts to go out of balance, disease will be the result—either disease of the mind, the body, or the spirit.

Accordingly, based on this practice, all that we have to do is to correct the imbalance and bring the officials as near to balance as we possibly can. Then the disease will disappear as nature ordains. How do we influence these officials? Well, each official in our body has a meridian (a pathway) going through it. Along the meridians flows *qi* energy. And it is this vital *qi* energy that enables each aspect to function.

Your officials can only function as well as *qi* energy will allow them to function. Along that meridian there are certain acupuncture points. Acupuncturists place needles in the points and influence the *qi* to balance the body so that the energy-vitality that the organs get is in balance. The use of acupuncture points influences the *qi* to make the officials function as near normal as one's nature allows.

Some meridians have as few as nine acupuncture points; on other meridians, there are over sixty. In the whole of the body, we have 365 points that influence the energy which flows to any one of our organs. The premise of acupuncture is that if we balance the officials, body, mind and spirit, the disease will disappear. A profound and bold statement, but this is at the core of the practice and theory of acupuncture.

The beauty of this approach to medical treatment is that we can pick up the distress signals as nature tells us, long before physical disease manifests. Almost immediately, nature tells us in many different ways when any organ starts to become unbalanced. Sending distress signals that say, "Hello, here is a warning signal. Pay attention to this," as if the body is signaling to preserve itself. For example, every time an organ in your body malfunctions, the color on your face changes.

Another way the body warns us relates to the sense of smell. If an organ becomes imbalanced in your body, your body emits an odor. A subtle odor is emitted from your body the minute an organ starts to malfunction. It is amazing that nature does this, but we must pay attention. You know that this is true when disease has fully manifested. If you smell correctly, you can smell that imbalance, that impending disease, before it manifests itself.

A third such signal is that as an organ becomes imbalanced, your emotions change. Another signal from nature is our body pulses. We have six pulses on one hand, and six pulses on the other. Each relates to one of the organs. The minute there is an imbalance in one of the organs, a skilled acupuncturist can feel it. This is what acupuncturists mean when they say they are "taking pulses." Another sign of an imbalance in an organ is in your voice. If you think about it, when you have a cold, get upset, stay out too late, you can hear that your voice changes. The organs, not you, control your voice. The same is true of each sensual signal.

Fortunately, we have these signals from the body. We have color, smell, our pulses; we have the emotions, and we have our voice. Normally, changes in these will take place over months and sometimes over a year before you actually get the disease. Nature is kind, and it tries to tell us there is a problem in many ways. We have to listen to our bodies to restore the balance of these organs and, thus, open the opportunity for healthy flow of energy and disease to disappear. There are many factors in reaching the goal of a balanced body, but when it is achieved, it is a beautiful thing—health and harmony.

There are five elements in this system of acupuncture: water, wood, fire, earth, and metal. We all contain bits of each, and depending on our individual bodies, we have a perfect balance and mix of these elements. The laws that are contained within the five elements are the Law of Mother/Child, the Law of Midday/Midnight, the Law of Husband/Wife, and the Law of Cure, and the Law of Five Elements. These are the unalterable natural laws. In acupuncture, by understanding these laws, we can understand more about ourselves and more easily understand the people around us.

Every disease has to follow The Law of the Cure if you are going to be healed and cured. The Law of the Cure is based on the premise that the disease has come from within your body to the outside; it will disappear in the reverse order. Therefore, to fully heal, you will need to go through the cancer and remove all the blockages that you have built up over time, peeling them back like an onion. This will allow you to follow The Law of the Cure and become healed—your energy will flow freely, without blockages, and enable your mind, spirit, and body to achieve the balance it needs to be well.

The acupuncturist tries to find the cause of the imbalance by studying the color, sound, odor, the pulses, the emotions, and the sound of the voice of his or her patient. That is going to help the acupuncturist discover the cause of the disease and the path that must be unblocked to begin to heal the patient. According to Chinese theory, most symptomatic approaches to diseases today do not cure but, instead, focus on suppressing the symptoms.

Every one of the elements is associated with an emotion. The element wood—the liver and gall bladder—is associated with the emotion of anger. Fire is associated with joy; earth, with sympathy; metal, with grief; and water, with fear. So there are five emotions that we each exhibit in a given set of circumstances.

We all are entitled to have strong emotions and share them with others. If the emotions are fitting, then, generally, it is a sign of health. If they are imbalanced, then it is a sign of disease. That is why we are never, ever simply physically sick. In the essence of acupuncture, mind, body, and spirit are one. To be healed, you must have a healthy body, mind, and spirit, you must have balance.

Jim still enjoys his acupuncture treatments, and in our minds there is no doubt that the combination of Western philosophy and Eastern philosophy in healing the body is a powerful one. We believe being open to acupuncture and other alternative healing arts only increases one's chances of full recovery.

NUTRITION AND DIET

God bless the roots! Body and soul are one.

—Theodore Roethke

The importance of reading and learning about certain food types became clear to us almost from the beginning of the healing process. Most of the learning we did on the subject of diet and nutrition came from books we purchased on-line and at the health food store. We also received advice from our doctors.

Some significant dietary changes we made are as follows:

- Switch from coffee to tea—black and green tea. *Why:* (a) green tea is potentially helpful in the treatment of prostate cancer; and (b) the caffeine in coffee can make you more anxious and stimulated than you should be.
- Replace all other oils and butters with olive oil. There are many types of olive oil, like extra-virgin, for spicing up bread, and regular olive oil to use in place of butter and other oils for cooking. (After a while you do not even notice it. I even use olive oil when making pancakes, but add a little vanilla for taste.) Canola oil is a backup to olive oil and has little flavor; use it in certain dishes that are overpowered by olive oil. *Why:* (a) Olive oil may reduce the risk of cancers of the colon, breast, prostate, and pancreas; (b) it reduces bad (LDL) cholesterol and increases good (HDL) cholesterol; and (c) it enhances absorption of lycopene.
- Reduce the amount of carbonated sodas by replacing them with water—loads of water. Jim drinks at least five to six 12-ounce servings of water per day. *Why:* Water is necessary because it transports waste products out of the body, carries nutrients around the body, and helps to regulate body temperature.

- We eliminated any prepared and/or packaged foods so I could monitor the organic nature of our foods and types of ingredients we were eating. *Why:* (a) Processed foods have many hidden cancer-causing agents, like preservatives, artificial sweeteners, and other harmful ingredients, and (b) they are often high in calories and fillers that have little or no nutritional value.

Overall, these changes were easy for us, more habit than anything else. Jim really never even seemed to notice—except for the coffee.

Because of the axiom "You are what you eat," Jim and I try to stay on the high protein/low fat side of the food chain. Based on feedback from our doctor, we watched closely to make sure Jim was getting enough protein by eating tuna, cheese, eggs, seafood, and other protein sources. The doctor was concerned that Jim may be eating too many carbohydrates and not enough protein. This was showing up in his blood work. For over a year after radiation, he had low hemoglobin counts, despite a full regimen of vitamins and herbs.

We believe our dietary changes must have had a positive effect, because many patients undergoing Jim's treatments gain ten to fifteen pounds. This was noted as a common side effect of the drugs. After three years of treatment and lots of meals, Jim still weighs the same. It takes discipline, but it is possible to go on hormone therapy and other treatments and not gain weight.

Today, the medical community has been able to correlate a specific factor in people's diets to many diseases. There seems to be anecdotal evidence of high fat intake as a cause of prostate cancer. However, since it is still a matter of debate, we have opted to focus on what can be done going forward rather than reflecting on past intake. Foods that have been identified as preventative and healing nature in regard to prostate cancer include tomatoes; fish, such as salmon; soy products; and green tea. Maybe they are not on your top-ten favorite foods list, but, as you will read later, they are foods for you to consider adding to your diet as a part of your healing plan.

You need not go overboard on the strictness of your diet, but be sensible and try to avoid foods high in fat, such as fried foods. Depending on the drugs you are taking, you may need to watch your total caloric intake to avoid gaining weight, especially if you are depressing the level of testosterone in your body.

To get some additional ideas about meals and foods to eat, you can purchase cookbooks made especially for sufferers of prostate cancers. Two top sellers include *Everyday Cooking With Dr. Dean Ornish: 150 Easy, Low-Fat, High-Flavor Recipes* by Dean Ornish, and *The Taste for Living Cookbook: Mike Milken's Favorite Recipes for Fighting Cancer* by Michael Milken. Ornish is a world-class researcher at UCSF. The recipes are easy to make, and most of the ingredients can be found in your local grocery store. The books can be found at most major bookstores or online.

Tomatoes; fish, such as salmon; soy products; and green tea contain ingredients known to be helpful in the prevention, containment, and treatment of prostate cancer. This list is not meant to be totally inclusive; it merely presents a few of the key foods you may want to consider as part of your diet.

FOODS FOR A HEALTHY PROSTATE

Food	Beneficial Component
Tomatoes/watermelon	Lycopene
Salmon/Halibut/Mackerel	Omega 3
Green tea	Omega 3
Soy products	Genestein

Tomatoes—Tomatoes of any kind are good, but they are even better when they are cooked, which increases the lycopene concentration. Lycopene is important in promoting a healthy prostate. Evidence of this has been cited in the *Prostate Newsletter* and by nutritionists such as Dr. Ornish. Additionally, Harvard Medical School, in Boston, did a study and determined that more than 50 percent of the men who ate tomatoes regularly had healthy prostates.

Salmon (and other fish rich in Omega 3, such as halibut and mackerel)—Fortunately, another great food for a healthy prostate is salmon. The reason for this is that salmon is rich in Omega 3. The reason Omega 3 is important is based on the outcome of a comparative study evaluating the diets of men in the United States and Japan. In Japan the incidence of prostate cancer was significantly lower than in the United States. As the researchers attempted to determine the reason for this, two specific items emerged. The first was the high presence of Omega 3 in all the fish Japanese men eat, and the second was green-tea consumption.

EPA (eicosapentaenoic acid) and DHA (docosahexaenoic acid) are the most important Omega-3 fatty acids. The table below lists the amount of EPA and DHA in certain fish and fish oils, plus their combined total.

OMEGA-3 FATTY ACIDS IN FISH AND FISH OILS

Fish oils / fish	Omega-3 Fatty Acids		Total Fish Oil (per 100 grams)
	EPA	DHA	
Salmon oil	8.8	11.1	19.9
Cod-liver oil	9.0	9.5	18.5
Atlantic mackerel	0.9	1.6	2.5
Pacific herring	1.0	0.7	1.7
Lake trout	0.5	1.1	1.6
Bluefin tuna	0.4	1.2	1.6
Sablefish	0.7	0.7	1.4
Chinook salmon	0.8	0.6	1.4
Lake whitefish	0.3	1.0	1.3
European sole	0.5	0.8	1.3
Sockeye salmon	0.5	0.7	1.2
Pink salmon	0.4	0.6	1.0
Pompano	0.2	0.4	0.6
Pacific oyster	0.4	0.2	0.6
Swordfish	1.0	0.5	0.6

Therefore, try to eat these fish two to three times a week, and add other products with Omega-3 to your diet, including fish-oil capsules. Avoid large amounts of cod-liver oil; it contains vitamins A and D, which can accumulate in toxic amounts in the body.

Fortunately, you can get fish fresh, frozen, and canned. Salmon can be used in the morning on a bagel, at lunch in a salad, or in the evening as an entrée. If and when you go out to dinner, fish is often on the menu as an appetizer or entrée. Live it up and try food that tastes good and is good for you, too!

Green tea—An ancient Japanese saying is, "If a man has no tea in him, he is incapable of understanding truth and beauty." Asian cultures have recognized the wonders of green tea for over 4,000 years. The tea's herbal qualities seem to dramatically reduce the incidence of cancer in people who drink it as a part of their normal diet. It has catechins that have been determined to be powerful natural antioxidants. In a recent study, prostate cells were mixed with testosterone and green-tea extract. The more green tea, the slower the growth of the prostate-cancer cells. Green tea's catechins lower the toxicity of certain carcinogens, thereby reducing their ability to cause cancer. Green tea contains a broad array of antioxidants—vitamin C, vitamin E, catechins, and bioflavonoids—that trap and destroy free radicals.

Green tea can be added to your diet in two ways. First, you can buy green tea as loose leaves or in tea bags. You can get the tea in larger grocery stores in the international foods section or in the tea section, and at health food stores or from a Chinese herbalist. The tea bags are better for simplicity, proper portioning, and portability, but when time permits, the leaves actually make a great pot of tea. The flavor of the tea takes a little getting used to, but before long you'll find yourself enjoying it. Steep green tea for 3 to 5 minutes, and then remove the bag for the best flavor and to avoid any bitter taste.

We find ourselves ordering it when we are out at dinner in Chinese, Japanese, or other Asian restaurants. Many of the coffee houses have it, and it is actually cheaper than a cup of coffee (which is not nearly as good for you). Again, this is a great way to incorporate green tea into your routine without a real change in your lifestyle.

Because of the overwhelmingly positive effects of green tea, you should not pass it up, but, realistically, finding it while traveling is not easy. To fit your lifestyle, you might want to go to an herbalist (or a vitamin store will do) and buy green tea–extract pills. There is no toxicity in green-tea pills and the amount of catechins is five to twenty times that of a cup of green tea. Take them every morning with your other pills, and it is done—one, two, three. This solution works great and might be worth a try. Many studies have concluded you need 300 to 1,000 milligrams of catechins to achieve health benefits. The average cup of green tea has 50 to 100 milligrams.

The only time not to drink green tea is during radiation treatment, when your doctor will most likely want you to stop taking all antioxidants. The reason for this is that radiation needs to attach to the free radicals in your body to effectively impact the future production of cancer cells. Antioxidants are crucial in lowering one's oxidative load, which has proven effective in fighting cancer (again, radiation patients may need to avoid antioxidants during radiation treatments). The antioxidant value in the table below is compared to the antioxidant power of vitamin E. Vitamin E is considered a highly useful antioxidant, so quercetin's value at 4.7 means it is especially effective. Renowned British professor and health author Catherine Rice Evans compiled this table.

FOODS HIGHEST IN ANTI-OXIDANTS

Antioxidant	Antioxidant Value	Food
Quercetin	4.7	Onions, apple skin, berries, black grapes, tea, broccoli
Cyanidin	4.4	Grapes, raspberries, strawberries
Lycopene	2.9	Tomatoes
Beta-carotene	1.9	Carrots, sweet potatoes, tomatoes, paprika, green vegetables
Taxifolin	1.9	Citrus fruits
Vitamin C	1.0	Fruits, vegetables
Vitamin E	1.0	Grains, nuts, oil

Soy—The last food, soy, may be newer to you than the others. You may have had soy in your miso soup at Japanese restaurants, or have tried it in a soy burger, but most Americans are not eating it as a part of their diet. However, here again the data is quite impressive. The Japanese eat a lot of soy products, and it turns out they contain genestein and other ingredients that have been proven to be helpful in prostate health and healing. Specific articles have been written and published in Dr. Dean Ornish's book *Healthy for Life,* in the *Prostate USTOO! Newsletter,* and by UCSF. There is no doubt, soy is one food not to miss when you have prostate cancer.

We do not recommend nonorganic soy, as it is heavily sprayed with pesticides that may cause cancer. There is a great deal of genetically modified soy (not labeled "organic") whose health effects are not yet known.

Soy milk is a good replacement for regular milk if you can get accustomed to the taste. It usually can be found on grocery shelves. Soy tofu has different textures, ranging from soft to hard. It can be added to foods you are quite used to making. Adding it to rice with soy sauce is very good and very easy. Including it in salad works, as well. You can buy soy nuts that are lightly salted, much less oily than peanuts, and have a great taste.

Alternatively, soy is available in daily pill form as a supplement. This works well, and it allows you to live a normal, hectic life without having to find a health food store for a tofu sandwich or some other option.

WHY SOY?

- Soy products offer a source of high-quality protein that is cholesterol free and low in saturated fats.
- Soy protein lowers triglycerides and LDL (bad cholesterol) without lowering HDL (good cholesterol).
- By substituting soy protein for meat, you may lessen the risk of kidney stones and osteoporosis.
- The instance of death from prostate cancer is low in those countries where soy represents a major protein source.
- Soy is rich in compounds called isoflavinoids. One of these, genistein, can block the growth of prostate cancer cells. At high levels, genistein kills prostate-cancer cells.

- One soy product, Ecogen 851, is reported to cause a positive response in 50 percent of prostate-cancer patients.
- Fermenting salted soybeans makes miso. This product is used in soups and stews, and can be used as a replacement for beef broth or chicken broth.
- The soybean produces five times as much protein per acre as wheat, ten times as much as dairy cattle, and twenty-five times as much as beef cattle.
- The soybean provides a source of high-quality protein, which is low in saturated fat and cholesterol free.
- Use soy products that have been processed with the traditional techniques used in Asia.

GENISTEIN VALUES IN SOY-BASED FOODS

Food	Genistein mg/100 grams,
Soy flakes	156
Soybean meal, whole	100
Soy flour	94
Soy nuts	94
Soybeans, roasted	87
Soybeans, green	73
Soy protein, textured	71
Soy isolate	56
Miso	52
Tofu, dry, spiced	42
Tempeh	40
Tofu, Kikkoman firm	31
Soybeans, dry, whole	20
Tempeh burger	20
Tofu	17

Anyone can add the foods mentioned in this chapter to their weekly diet, but accept it takes time to adjust to these items if they are not currently a part of your diet. Add them one by one so you don't make yourself believe you are changing everything you eat because of prostate cancer. You will most likely be more successful if you slowly modify your diet, not radically alter it in a day. You can happily use these ingredients in your normal diet if you put them on your shopping list, experiment with the foods, and keep an open mind. If you use tomatoes, salmon (or similar fish), and soy three times a week as an entrée or a part of your meals, you are well on your way to bringing these vital foods into your life. You can change your diet without too much hassle.

To help you get started with ideas on how you can use tomatoes, fish, soy, and green tea, here are a few recipes you might like to try. Think of this part of the healing process as a way to expose yourself to new flavors and tastes.

Tomato-Mushroom Sauce w/Linguine

2–3 tablespoons olive oil
1 onion (chopped fine)
6–8 mushrooms (chopped)
2–3 cloves of garlic (fresh)
1 can whole tomatoes or 8 fresh tomatoes chopped
1 can tomato paste (6 oz.)
2 teaspoons basil
1 teaspoon oregano
1 teaspoon parsley
Salt and pepper, to taste

Place oil in pan and heat. Add onion to the pan and cook until tender. Add mushrooms and garlic. Cook until soft. Add tomatoes, tomato paste, basil, oregano, parsley, salt and pepper. Bring to a boil, and then simmer for 60 minutes. Serve over precooked linguine.

Salmon Filets with Dill Sauce

2–4 salmon filets (approximately 6 ounces each)
1–1½ cups of milk
6 tablespoons honey Dijon mustard
2 tablespoons sour cream
Fresh dill, chopped
1 lemon, cut in wedges for garnish

Soak salmon filets in milk for three to four hours—the longer, the more tender. Place ¾ inches water in a fish steamer, and bring to a boil. (If you don't have a fish steamer, use a frying pan with a lid). Alternative: Wrap salmon tightly in aluminum foil; place in pan, with foil opening above the waterline. Poach for about 15–20 minutes, depending on filet. Fish should be pink-orange and flaky. Do not overcook.

Dill Sauce–

Combine honey Dijon mustard, sour cream, and chopped dill. Mix.

Serve salmon with lemon wedges and sauce on the side.

Green-Tea Ice Cubes

3 bags green tea
3 cups of boiling water

Boil water, and add tea bags; remove from heat. Steep for 5 minutes, and then remove bags. Place tea in ice-cube tray, and freeze. Add two or three cubes to cold drinks, regular iced tea, or drinks.

Soy Rice

2 tablespoons olive or canola oil
3 scallions, chopped
4–6 ounces tofu; chopped into ½-inch squares
2 eggs
2 cups just-cooked brown rice
1–3 tablespoons soy sauce, to taste
Salt and pepper, to taste

Heat oil, add chopped scallions, and soy sauce; sauté. In a small bowl, mix eggs. Remove scallions from pan, and scramble eggs. As they are finishing, add rice, soy sauce, salt, and pepper. Mix thoroughly. Then add tofu and scallion, mix, and serve with extra soy sauce on the side. Makes 2–3 portions.

The National Cancer Institute recommends a low-fat diet, including plenty of fruits, vegetables, and whole grains, to reduce the risk of all types of cancer. Evidence suggests that a high-fat diet contributes to the risk of prostate cancer. This, however, is inconsistent with some studies indicating that dietary fat is not a major risk factor for prostate cancer. Clinical trials are underway to study whether a low-fat, high-fiber diet that is high in soy, fruits, vegetables, green tea, and vitamin E will reduce incidence of prostate cancer. Keep your eyes open for more data on diet and prostate cancer. This type of research is still only in its nascent stage.

Detox Programs

As we started to tell friends that Jim had prostate cancer, they were often eager to give us advice based on their experiences or those of others they knew. The idea of detoxing/fasting was introduced to us in the second month of Jim's treatment. We decided to explore this avenue primarily because of input from one of our friends. She had been fasting throughout her life and believed it was one of the reasons she was so vibrant and healthy. Additionally, another friend of hers with advanced cancer had been treating her illness with Western medicine and fasting and had been cancer free for over five years.

In Western history, fasting has long been a spiritual and physical means to purification. Both Moses and Jesus fasted for forty days; Socrates and Plato fasted for ten-day stretches prior to beginning major writing works. Fasting gives the entire digestive system, including the stomach, intestines, pancreas, gall bladder, and liver a chance to rest. Abstaining from food increases the release of toxins from the colon, liver, kidneys, bladder, lungs, sinuses, and skin. Some fasting experts believe that fasting boosts the immune system. There are studies in which rats who had a restricted food intake had fewer instances of cancer and lived longer than rats on a regular diet.

The belief is that fasting encourages us to follow our true nature by removing the noise and activity of eating and digesting food from the body. During a detox program, self-realization and the desire for change are often stimulated; many people review aspects of their lives and end up questioning their relationships, careers, healing, and plans for the future. You may feel spiritually awakened, with greater mental and emotional clarity. While fasting, people often confront and discuss their problems. Apparently, a feeling of liberation and a determination to eliminate obstacles and negative aspects of one's life are common to the experience.

As usual, we went on a mission and bought five books on diet and fasting. We ended up with one main guide, plus some improvisations, that fit our lifestyle. It was the first time in my life we had purchased this type of material. Before, we had not felt the need to explore these types of alternative practices, but now we were willing to try many new things. The detox experience was probably one of the most intense activities we undertook as a couple. It was a complete body detoxing via body cleansing and fasting. From my perspective, this was the one of the most far-out healing activities we did.

Before we could even consider starting this option, we discussed it with our doctor and made sure he was okay with the idea. In Jim's case, we felt it was important to try a detox program as a way to support his body through the treatment process. We opted to try an initial ten-day detox in June, four weeks prior to Jim's first radiation treatment. We thought this made sense because, ideally, he would start radiation with his body in as healthy a state as possible.

Detoxing was very difficult for me, but I did it because it was an active way to show my support for Jim and to take time to purge myself of some of the effects of our struggle. It was a way for me to experience the idea of being uncomfortable during Jim's healing process. It helped me be more understanding about feeling weak and what his body must be going through on a daily basis.

Our first detox program went on for ten long, long days. Talk about getting in touch with your body! It included a weeklong detox period and three days of entry and exit from the experience. The fasting portion included about thirty-six hours of complete fasting. The first few days were very difficult. I was hungry and irritable, and I wanted my Diet Pepsi. I had a headache on days two and three; Jim had a headache on day two from caffeine withdrawal. But, as if a great magic wand passed over us, by the fourth day we had adjusted to no caffeine and no sugar. Days four and five passed slowly, but they did pass. On day six into the experience—the day of the total fast—we took the easy way out: a double feature. We went to the movies and sat through two films. Before we knew it the day was over. By this time in the fast, believe it or not, we were really not hungry any more. Our bodies had started to operate on liquids and we felt great.

By the end of the detox period, we felt spiritually awakened and had greater mental and emotional clarity. The clutter in our minds was reduced, and we felt closer to our real selves and to God. We slept better, probably because we had no food to power our bodies. While fasting, we confronted and discussed problems that had been buried for years. This feeling of liberation and the determination to eliminate obstacles and negative aspects of one's life are allegedly not unusual during detox. One of the other side effects is that you really do feel your body cleansing itself. My bowel movements changed significantly. My body perspiration was different, and during my workouts I broke into a sweat much faster. I had a lot more open time, because the two to three hours normally spent engaged in mealtime, preparation, and cleanup were no longer required.

Selecting ten consecutive days on our calendar when we were not engaged in a hectic physical or mental schedule was vital to our success. We found that starting on Monday was ideal, because the most difficult days of total fasting take place on days six and seven. This made us choose Saturday and Sunday, when life was just a bit slower for those days.

Jim and I did another ten-day detox in October, after the radiation therapy was over. This felt like a rite of passage. After three years of treatment and the final hormone-therapy shot, we waited three months to do our last full-length detox. It was as if the fasting was required for us to go full circle through the entire healing process. Quite frankly, I am not sure whether detoxing made a significant difference in Jim's healing success. I do know it made us feel we were doing everything possible to create a healing environment for Jim's body and immune system. It gave our bodies a rest, and both of us were sorely in need of rest.

We all are guilty of overindulging and polluting our bodies from time to time. The whole concept of detoxing, or fasting, is to give your body a rest by allowing it to rid itself of as many toxins as possible. The process can be done at anytime prior to, during, or after specific Western medical treatments like radiation therapy and surgery.

The first rule of detoxing is to fast only if you are feeling healthy. Always consult your doctor first. If you are taking any medications, be sure to check with your physician before embarking on the detox program. Many drugs behave differently on an empty stomach. It is not recommended to fast during a period in your life when you have many physical or mental demands. Each person and situation is unique. It is best to regard a fasting period as a time of reflection and rest. In many religious practices, holy fast days are usually linked to prayer and meditation.

Spring, for example, is a natural time to flush the toxins that have been building up all winter long. According to Chinese medicine, the transition between the seasons is considered to be about ten days before and after the equinox or solstice. Following a detox program twice a year would probably make you a hardcore detox person. Not only will your digestive system benefit, but you'll also notice other changes. During a fast you should consume at least eight six-ounce glasses of water and keep physical activity to a minimum.

Listed next are examples of simple detox/fasting programs that you can try. The first time is probably the most difficult, because you may never have experienced this type of thing before. But after you do it once, it is not that hard the second time around.

ONE-DAY DETOX

Breakfast

1 large glass freshly squeezed orange, apple, or grapefruit juice

Mid Morning Snack

1 cup herbal tea with a small amount of honey or lemon

Lunch and Dinner

1 large glass fresh vegetable juice

NOTE: No food after 6 P.M. Drink at least eight to twelve 6-ounce glasses of spring water during the day. Try to do a one-day detox for the first time on a weekend.

THREE-DAY JUICE DETOX/FAST

JUICE FLUSH

½ cup fresh orange or apple juice

1 thin strip of ginger, chopped

2 cloves garlic, chopped

8 ounces of spring water

Mix all the ingredients together, and enjoy! Drink two glasses of this mixture each day, one before 10 A.M. and one before 3 P.M.

Midday Snack

1 cup freshly squeezed vegetable juice

Note: No juice after 6 P.M Drink at least eight to twelve 6-ounce glasses of spring water daily and as much chamomile tea, peppermint tea, or water as desired.

With all fasts and detox programs, break them slowly by introducing additional juices, raw fruits, and vegetables the day after the fast is completed. This will allow your body to adjust to food reentering into your system. After completing the program, you should have energy and enthusiasm to spare. During this period in your life, choose to be alone or with your partner (or any person who is going through the process with you) as much as possible. Fellow fasters have reported closer feelings to their spiritual center and a desire to pray. If this happens, go with your desire. Be conscious of new feelings; allow yourself to be led by your soul and inspiration. Use this time to simplify your life. If the weather is accommodating, spend as much time as possible outdoors in the sunshine, taking leisurely walks and appreciating nature.

Working is very difficult during the time of detoxing, so consider it only if you can slow down your schedule dramatically or, ideally, take time off work. We did work, but only from our home office. We did not attempt to travel or socialize.

EXERCISE

To keep a body in good health is a duty. . . . Otherwise we shall not be able to keep our mind strong and clear.

—Buddha

Before cancer, Jim and I had incorporated regular exercise into our lives. After the diagnosis, however, Jim became much more devoted to it. He worked out daily as a part of his healing routine, and this did wonders for him in many ways. It relieved his stress, it gave him energy to make it through the treatments, and it gave him an amazingly positive outlook. Jim used exercise as a time for self-healing, a release of all the negative and poisonous thoughts he had, and to build up a sweat to keep him strong and healthy.

To assist Jim initially, we hired a trainer: James, a wonderful young man who was studying to become a chiropractor and already certified to teach physical-fitness training. His young, healthy attitude and firm commitment to keeping Jim strong was perfect support. The drugs Jim was on caused his muscle mass to decrease and his bone mass to weaken. Therefore, exercise was important to ensure that his body would continue to be strong after recovery. When he was off the drugs, Jim wanted to reduce the risk of any long-term bone or muscle loss due to prolonged physical weakness from the treatments.

Jim worked out with James twice a week for six weeks just prior to the start of his treatment plan. During radiation treatment, Jim continued under James's instruction with weights and stretching once a week. He also worked out with weights on his own two to three additional days a week. The workouts required about one hour with weights and thirty to forty minutes of aerobic exercise, sit-ups, and other intensive activities, such as running on the treadmill.

To this day, Jim continues his weight training and aerobic exercise. He runs three to four miles each day. He does his sit-ups everyday and is dedicated to weight training and stretching four to six times per week, depending on his workout plans. All of this time spent is a healthy, healing escape. It allows his body to be number one in his life. A critical success factor for Jim is that he does not allow anyone, any appointment, or any travel plans to prevent his working out. It is the first thing he does in the morning, besides taking his Fosomax pill and drinking his tea. Jim places his body first, and this sends the positive signal to his mind and soul that he is working hard at healing and curing.

Less than one month after Jim ended three years of hormone therapy, he ran his first half-marathon—13.6 miles up a mountain at Napa State Park, in Napa, California. We did this with our daughter and some of her childhood friends. It was a momentous time that gave us an appropriate metaphor for this critical stage in the treatment of prostate cancer. Fighting cancer is a full marathon and we have only gone a little over halfway, but we are still in the race.

Jim and I passionately believe that exercise was a significant factor in his recovery. When Jim exercises, there is no outside noise, no invasion of drugs, but only the soul and the body healing together. The soul asks the body: "Why have you betrayed me? I thought I was doing okay." And the body, through exercise to gain strength, responds: "Not always. You took me for granted. I am vulnerable. I am fragile, and I can be broken. Please take care of me. Feed me with positive thoughts, healthful foods, and plenty of water, and nurture me with rest, love, and healing drugs. I will do my best to be a good body. Now, you do your best to be a happy soul with positive mental energy." Couldn't a body be saying this by crying out with such disease? I believe body, mind, and soul work together to begin the miraculous process of healing, the three working in unison to the beat of a runner's pace, a biker's cadence, or a hiker's step.

Here is a humorous bit of writing found on the Internet, about exercise, that you might appreciate.

TO EXERCISE, OR NOT TO EXERCISE

1. It is well documented that for every mile you jog, you add one minute to your life. This enables you, at age 85, to spend an additional five months in a nursing home at $5,000 per month.
2. My grandmother started walking five miles a day when she was sixty. She is now ninety-seven, and we don't know where she is.

3. I would only take up jogging so I could hear heavy breathing again.
4. I joined a health club last year, and spent about $400—haven't lost a pound. Apparently you have to show up.
5. I have to exercise early in the morning, before my brain figures out what I am doing.
6. I don't exercise at all. If God meant us to touch our toes, he would have put them further up our body.
7. I like long walks, especially when they are taken by people who annoy me.
8. I have flabby thighs, but fortunately my stomach covers them.
9. The advantage of exercising every day is that you die healthier.
10. And last, but not least, I don't jog—it makes the ice jump right out of my glass.

During thirty minutes or more of exercise, you not only expend calories, but also burn fat, lower cholesterol levels, build muscle and bone, and improve your mental health. Most books on health tell you to exercise about three hours a week to maintain a healthy body. It helps you in many ways—sleeping, weight control, stamina, strength, mental ability, and on and on.

One of the most important aspects of exercise is that it makes you feel good. One of the best ways exercise helps cancer patients is by letting them escape negative thoughts by turning those thoughts into positive energy. Exercise allows you to escape to a place where you are alone, with only your mind and body interacting with each other. Whether it is at the gym, during running, or on the seat of a bicycle, exercise helps you escape. For the time you are involved in the exercise, even though your mind may be racing at first, by the middle to the end of the workout you are focused on getting through it and enjoying the sense of accomplishment. You have set a goal for yourself, and in thirty minutes each day, you can achieve it.

Weight training is important as a supplement to aerobic exercise, because many prostate-cancer treatments have side effects that can weaken bones and deteriorate muscle mass. It is a good idea to initiate a weight-training plan at the same time or right after you undergo your treatments. Your doctor and a professional trainer will give you advice based on your specific situation. Your weight-training plan should include all major muscle groups, such as those in your arms, legs, back, stomach, and shoulders.

You might want to consider hiring a personal trainer if this is all new to you. One can usually be found at local fitness centers and can customize a workout plan just for you. If you do not have the funds for a trainer, you can go to the library and check out books, DVDs, and videos on weight training. By purchasing a couple of sets of free weights and resistance tools, you can strengthen and train your body in the privacy of your home.

VITAMINS AND HERBS

Ritual is the technique for giving life.

—Thomas Peters and Robert Waterman, Jr.

Jim and I discussed alternative therapy as part of exploring Eastern options in addition to Western ones. He said he was open to the idea, and I was off like a rocket to investigate. After consulting with one of my Hawaiian friends who was a huge believer in alternative medicine, she referred me to a Chinese herbalist. We later found another practitioner in the San Francisco area to follow her initial treatments.

The Hawaiian herbalist's storefront was not well marked. In fact, I would have walked right by it if I didn't have the address and street number. There was no big sign. This was the type of practitioner you found through word-of-mouth and the Chinese community. The shop was very plain inside. There was a large counter—the sort you used to see at a general store—and there was only a dry-measure scale on it—no cash register, no items to get you to buy impulsively at the last minute, only the scale and sheets of brown paper neatly stacked one on top of each other.

When I entered, I caught an immediate whiff of medicine, one with an outdoor type of aroma that was different than anything I had ever smelled before. It was unusual and made me think I was in a place where I was going to be exposed to products I had never heard of before. Behind the counter, shelves made of small wooden boxes lined the walls almost to the ceiling. They looked like one massive mailbox with hundreds of drawers. On each box there was a white index card in a cardholder with neat Chinese characters on it. From what I could tell, each one looked different, but I was not knowledgeable enough to know and not comfortable enough to ask. Between the shelves there was a doorway that led to a large room. In there, I saw a table that was used for acupuncture, and more space dedicated to the ancient art of herbs.

Our Hawaiian herbalist was a woman trained in China. By the looks I received, I felt I was one of the few female Caucasians to enter her clinical store. She, however, was very understanding and made me feel comfortable. She asked for details about Jim— his age, his weight, overall health, how long he had known about the cancer, and how serious it was. Referring to the handwritten notes she took while I answered her questions, she asked me to sit down and told me it would be ten to fifteen minutes while she blended the herbs. I sat there with the smell of dried twigs and earth, and waited.

When the herbalist was finished, she gave me a series of capsules the contents of which had just been mixed together. Additionally, she gave me liquid shot bottles of what I learned were astragalus plus a mixture for tea. Jim was to drink it at least once a day and take the pills three times a day. I asked her what the herbs were. Somehow I felt very safe with this herbalist, but I was curious about the ingredients. She told me about them all, and off I went feeling like I was really helping Jim.

I bought several books on herbs and vitamins and shared with Jim information on the herbs he was taking. This made us feel good too, knowing that the herbs she discussed were right there in a herbal reference book as viable treatments for prostate cancer. We also found that there are some potent vitamins to take for prostate cancer.

The Ritual of Herbs

Jim began a ritual of daily herbs and vitamins and still religiously takes an updated version of them today. While it may seem simple to start, keeping track of what herbs and drugs need to be taken each day can be challenging. We decided to create pre-prepared packages for Jim. It made it easy for him to take the medication, and it made it easy for me to make sure he was getting these important supplements. On Saturday, I would usually prepare a twenty-one-day batch of individual daily dosages of vitamins and herbs. That way we could keep track of our supplies and reorder prior to the next batch preparation. Jim found Ziploc Baggies worked best to hold all of the pills. I would place twenty-one of them on the table and make three rows with seven piles each of vitamins and herbs. During that time, I would fill my mind with positive thoughts about how those herbs and vitamins were helping to heal and cure him. I would stop for a moment and be thankful for these herbs that could make his body and immune system strong.

Jim developed a ritual of healing that mixed the Chinese herbs and vitamins with the "four horsemen" (the drugs from our Western treatment plan: Casodex, Fosomax, and Proscar, plus Synthroid, a drug needed for a slow thyroid). As Jim would take these pills every morning he would consciously thank God for letting his body take in the medicine and for healing him. He keeps the pills in a special bowl right next to the refrigerator in the kitchen. In with the drugs is a red chocolate heart I put there over three years ago to remind him to take the drugs with love in his heart and mind. While it may not seem important, I believe this positive attitude toward the experience and being active in the healing process was critical for Jim's success. He knew how important these drugs were to his well-being, and the daily ritual helped to reinforce this. From that point forward, Jim made sure that he sat down right before breakfast, grabbed a water bottle from the fridge, and methodically emptied the bag of herbs and vitamins plus his other pills from the doctor. With a few pills at a time, he purposefully took into his body his formula for healing.

Once we moved to San Francisco for our treatment plan at UCSF, we were in search of a new herbalist. We were referred to Michael Broffman, who had studied homeopathic healing. He was also very knowledgeable about vitamins. This was helpful because, while I had started to give Jim a multivitamin, selenium, and vitamin E, there was much more that could and should be done based upon his Western treatment plan.

Michael ran Pine Street Benevolent Chinese Center in San Anselmo, across the bay from San Francisco. Just like a Western doctor, Michael wanted Jim's full history and verbally reviewed the details of his past for over an hour. We paid for his services on the initial visit, just as you would any Western doctor; the only difference is this type of visit is not covered by insurance. His diagnosis and recommended treatment was exceedingly thorough and well worth the expense. He was very knowledgeable about the power of herbs and vitamins. He spelled out a detailed daily regime for Jim, based on his upcoming radiation therapy. The regime called for taking pills three times per day. We found this impossible to execute but we modified it and Jim took the herbs and vitamins once or sometimes twice a day.

Michael changed Jim's prescription four times throughout his treatment: the first time prior to radiation, then during radiation, then post-radiation (for two and a half years), and finally after Jim was off all the cancer treating drugs. This is important, to be sensitive to what phase of healing your body is in and when you may need different herbs and vitamins. Even though Jim is currently off his Western medicine and drugs, he still takes all his adjusted regimen of herbs and vitamins.

Preradiation Treatment

The Chinese herbs included astragulus, milk thistle, green-tea supplements (vitamin E, vitamin C, and selenium), saw palmetto, licorice, calcium, shark cartilage, a complete multivitamin, and a mushroom complex. This combination of herbs and vitamins was designed to help the tumor shrink and aid the body's immune system to overcome the prostate cancer.

During Jim's radiation treatment, our radial oncologist recommended that Jim stop taking the antioxidants. We did not want to reduce the radiation effect on cancer cells. Jim only took saw palmetto, licorice, milk thistle, mushroom complex, and T-cell compound. While the effect of the herb regime is unclear, Jim's result from radiation was exceedingly successful. His PSA went from 1.1 to below .02 and he did not have the PSA bump that can occur after radiation. We believe that the combination of the vitamins and herbs, diet, exercise, and participation in support groups helped Jim to accomplish this amazing result.

After radiation, Jim went back to an aggressive schedule of herbs and vitamins, including organic soy essentials (with genistein, daidzein, and beta-glucans), calcium with magnesium, conjugated linoleic acid, vitamin C, vitamin E, a powerful multivitamin, selenium, saw palmetto, milk thistle, T-cell builder, inisotol, mushroom complex, omega 3, and green-tea supplements. This may seem like a lot of herbs and vitamins, but we believe all the pieces of Jim's healing plan have worked together for a positive outcome. Jim continues to take herbs and vitamins daily, and checks in with his herbalist for an assessment on a regular basis.

Western medical doctors are not always willing to discuss the use of herbs and vitamins for prostate cancer, but we learned that it is an area that you can take control of yourself through books, resource centers, and experts. Our UCSF doctors felt that such additional treatments were potentially beneficial. They made us feel that our interdisciplinary approach to healing and curing was the right one. They were supportive and not threatened by alternative medicine, which was exciting to us.

In terms of your time, energy, and choices in dealing with cancer, think of herbs and vitamins as one way you can personally extend your healing effort. If you are interested in this kind of treatment, please see a professional herbalist or nutritionist for advice. The herbs and vitamins we discuss here may not be exactly right for you; however, including some form of vitamin and herbal component in your treatment plan can be a powerful complement to the drugs you are getting from your doctor.

Powerful Vitamins

To give you insight into the strength of a few of the most important vitamins and herbs here are the vitamins that kept coming up in our research: omega 3, genestein, vitamin E, selenium, vitamin C, and a combination of zinc, calcium, and magnesium. There are literally thousands of vitamins and herbs to consider, and a visit to a trained herbalist is key to creating the best formula for you. Asking your doctor directly about this subject will be helpful as well. He or she may have certain regimens for you to follow.

Another topic often discussed was organic herbs and vitamins. Going out of your way to find organic sources is promoted by a variety of resources. We opted to buy organic, but you will have to decide what is best for your treatment plan.

Omega 3

Omega 3 is a polyunsaturated, highly unstable fat. Flaxseed oil has the highest concentration of omega 3 of all vegetable oils. Other vegetable oils that contain omega 3 are canola and soy oil. A regular dose of fresh flaxseed or omega 3 pills is best. Flaxseed oil is highly susceptible to going rancid if not refrigerated.

Omega 3 is an essential fatty acid that is a precursor for prostaglandin production. Prostaglandins are an important group of hormonelike chemicals that regulate almost every major body function, such as the immune system, blood pressure, and fluid retention. These chemicals can be found naturally in salmon, mackerel, and halibut.

Selenium

I often tell men that if they take no other vitamins, make sure that selenium and vitamin E are part of their regimen. Selenium is an important micronutrient, an essential trace element. Selenium added in trace amounts protects against a wide variety of carcinogens. Additionally, there is research indicating that selenium may have potential as a chemotherapeutic agent for treating cancer.

A study by Dr. Schranzer analyzed blood-bank data from various countries and demonstrated that there is a statistical relationship between levels of selenium in the body and their impact on cancer. Countries with lower levels of selenium had higher levels of cancers of the breast, colon, prostate, and lung. There is an inverse relationship between selenium availability and total cancer mortality in men and women. The recommended dosage is 200 milligrams in pill form to be taken daily.

Selenium	High doses of selenium can cause illness and, in extreme cases, death. 200-mcg/day is the suggested maximum from natural diet. If you have questions about selenium levels in your region, limit the daily selenium dose to less than 50 mcg/day.

Vitamin E

Vitamin E is a strong antioxidant and possesses anticancer activity both alone and in combination with other anticancer nutrients. Vitamin E helps the immune system operate at an optimum level. It has been shown that vitamin E and selenium have synergistic effects: Selenium enhances vitamin E's effectiveness.

The ability of antioxidant nutrients to boost the immune system and fight cancer is greater when they work together. Clinical trials now underway are examining the preventative benefits of vitamin E and selenium, both separately and in combination.

In *Eating Your Way to Better Health* by Dr. Charles Myers, a scientific study links increases in vitamin E consumption to a decreased death rate from cancer. Prostate cancer cells produce hydrogen peroxide and oxidants, and vitamin E lessens the damage that these oxidants cause to genetic material in the cell. Presumably, this slows the cancer cells' ability to mutate and invade other tissues. There is evidence that vitamin E kills prostate cancer cells by a unique mechanism. All cells have the ability to commit suicide, even cancer cells. It appears that vitamin E activates proteins (like Fas) called "death receptors," and the cancer cell destroys itself. These antioxidants help control growth and function of the prostate epithelial cells (the prostate lining). Having sufficient amounts of these nutrients in your diet may help prevent prostate cancer.

In a recent study of 29,000 male smokers, those who took 50 milligrams per day of vitamin E in the form of alpha-tocopherol (the equivalent of 50 IU of vitamin E) for five to eight years had thirty-two percent fewer cases of prostate cancer and forty-one percent fewer deaths from prostate cancer than those taking a placebo. New studies indicate that either gamma-tocopheral or delta-tocotrienal may be even more effective than alpha-tocopherol against cancer cells. In a ten-year study of more that 900 male skin-cancer patients, those who took a daily tablet containing 200 micrograms of selenium in the form of brewer's yeast for four-and-a-half-years had an almost two-thirds lower incidence of prostate cancer six years later, compared with those who took a placebo.

Ideal dosage is 400 to 800 IU of mycelized vitamin E daily, based on the data we read. Ideally, use the natural rather than the synthetic form of vitamin E. Food sources of vitamin E include fortified cereals, tomatoes, and nuts. Selenium is found mainly in brewer's yeast, grains, meat, and fish.

Vitamin C

Vitamin C is essential for the immune system to function effectively. Cells called NK (natural killer) cells kill abnormal cells. NK cells are active only if they contain relatively large amounts of vitamin C. The recommended dosage ranges from 500 milligrams to 1,000 milligrams and can be taken in pill or chewable form.

Daily supplementation of vitamin C has been shown to decrease the amount of chromosome damage induced in lymphocytes, abolish the secretion of stress hormones, and help people with low-back pain and arthritis, due to its antioxidant effects.

<table>
<tr><td>Vitamin C</td><td>Vitamin C does not prevent prostate cancer from developing.
Note: High doses of Vitamin C can cause kidney stones.
Vitamin C doses of 500–1,000 mg. are recommended by the FDA.</td></tr>
</table>

Soy

As mentioned earlier, soy is vital in your diet as a food or supplement. Evidence from over forty studies suggests that a diet rich in soy protein plays a substantial role in the promotion of healthy prostate function. In fact, the areas of highest soy consumption exhibit the lowest mortality rates from prostate cancer. Based on research done by Dr. Dean Ornish and others, one is encouraged to eat this base food of a Japanese diet enhanced in the United States by a vitamin supplement. The key ingredients of soy are genestein and daidzein plus beta-glucans. The recommended amounts are around 8 milligrams to 10 milligrams of genestein and daidzein and 25 milligrams to 30 milligrams of beta-glucans. Soy is believed to be very helpful in the total health of the prostate.

Zinc, Calcium, and Magnesium

The last important mineral is a combination of zinc, magnesium, and calcium, meant to support the bones, muscles, and immune system. Calcium and magnesium in balance are needed for proper conduction of electrical impulses in nerves and muscles. Taken with zinc, they are mild neuromuscular relaxants, promoting sleep at bedtime and protecting the immune system. Hormone therapy causes a loss of muscle and bone mass and must be counterbalanced with proper nutrition and vitamins.

Vitamins and herbs are a part of our life today, and we will continue to have them as supplements to our daily diet. The data on their effectiveness is growing all the time, and there is the possibility for other breakthroughs. Intentionally, we have stayed away from discussing those herbs and vitamins about whose medical value we could not find evidence to support

BUILDING YOUR NETWORK

Surround yourself with people who respect and treat you well.

—Claudia Black

Taking inventory of strong relationships in his life is something that Jim naturally did soon after he was diagnosed with cancer. "Who is going to be there for me?" is an important question that you, too, might find yourself asking.

Cancer causes you to think deeply about the people in your life. As you enter the implementation phase of your treatment, you might begin to realize that it is a journey you do not want to undertake alone. You may begin to accept things for what they are—not easy, but realistic. You may be asking many questions and experiencing many doubts, fears, and anxieties. But I believe that one of the best ways to help you get through the entire healing process is to learn from others. You will be able to gather strength and love from them to help you through the process.

By building a network of your family, friends, other cancer patients, professional doctors and practitioners, you can accomplish much more with them on your side than with tackling the illness all on your own. In addition to your family and friends, support can take many forms: conferences, seminars, self-help sessions, and support groups. Others can offer advice, listen, share experiences, and more. Each person can give a part of themselves and their experience to you if you allow yourself to open up to him or her.

Women are usually more comfortable reaching out to another woman, a friend, or an informal acquaintance to talk about issues that trouble them. Men have a tendency to keep their emotions bottled up inside. But when you have a life-threatening disease, when you are facing this monumental challenge of your life in which you are not in control, you may need to think differently about reaching out to others for their support. In particular, the input of those in the same situation as you can be crucial to your healing process. For Jim and I, support from family, friends, and other cancer patients with the same disease has been intrinsic to Jim's healing process.

Family

Telling our family about Jim's cancer was one of the most difficult steps for us, because neither of us knew exactly what to say. All of our immediate and extended family was spread throughout the United States. Our children are adults in their twenties. Initially we thought we would visit them in person to tell them the news, but then Jim decided it would be better to tell them sooner and over the phone. Jim decided to be very general with our kids about the cancer. There were vast amounts we didn't know in terms of the long-term prognosis, and he decided it would be best to keep it at high level and not try to get involved in the details of the treatments and the risks. Even during illness, your role as father and protector is as important as ever. Rather than having your children experience fear, uncertainty, and thoughts of death, it is natural to try to shield them from this reality. Concurrently, there is a fear of admitting to them the anxieties and inner struggles of your mortality. It is a time of tough love for all.

The conversations we had with our children were not nearly as stressful for us as was planning a trip and building up all the anxiety of telling them in person. After a few minutes of general catching up about their lives, Jim shared with them that he had prostate cancer. *Cancer* was a word they had heard before from their father because he had had basal-cell skin cancer at one time. This time, the cancer was in a different place—and much more severe.

Both children had the same initial reaction: disbelief. Jim, as father and consoler, kept the conversation moving, telling them he was seeing great doctors and he was very confident of a positive outcome. They had a few questions, but throughout the thousand days of treatment, their discussions with Jim about his cancer were minimal. We established a "don't ask, don't tell" situation, and that seemed to work best for us.

In a totally different situation, after about a year into the treatment, Jim received a call from a family member of a friend with prostate cancer. Two of the friend's three children wanted to meet with us to learn as much as they could about the disease and how it would affect their father and them. When we met them, we could tell they were anxious and eager to learn. They asked us questions about UCSF, the hospital experience, radiation, what the PSA score really meant, and on and on. After about two hours of answering all the questions we could, we recommended they explore other resources, like the UCSF Resource Center, a place filled with a wealth of knowledge. They left with a sense of hope for their dad. As a follow up, Jim received a beautiful, heartfelt phone call from his friend thanking him for taking the time to do this. In our own way, helping another family cope with this situation helped us, too. We were able to review all the steps that we went through, such as fear, anger, denial, and depression, and then emerge with a sense of hope, unity of body and mind, and an amazing appreciation for the beauty in life.

Just as each individual is different, the ways that children accept, process, and live with illness in the family are unique. There are no right or wrong ways here, only knowing that you are trying to do your best based on what you know at that moment. It is a time to let go and release the "old tapes" we replay about family and relationships and to realize that the only change we can make is to reprocess history and release past pain to allow for future healing and growing. The only control one has is to deal with the present and plan for the future with a resolve to build, nurture, and retain healthy relationships with family and friends.

Of course, when our children first learned of Jim's illness, we all felt a great deal of sadness and fear. They wanted to know what prostate cancer was and how serious it was, but future conversations moved beyond the disease to what was happening in their lives. This approach seemed to work very well for Jim and for our kids.

Because Jim's father had prostate cancer, he was very aware of the disease and the potential outcomes. He was very helpful to Jim because he had been through surgery five years earlier and had no long-term side effects. However, in the last two years he went onto hormone therapy as well. Jim was able to share his stories with his dad about hot flashes and the other side effects. This experience brought the two of them closer. There was a real sense of love and caring between them that emerged as they both genuinely opened up to their emotions about their health and their relationship.

Many other experiences happened to our family as we were living through prostate cancer. Life on all levels did continue to move on and other events did occur that helped us to keep everything in perspective. Throughout the years we lost my grandfather; we placed Jim's mom, who had Alzheimer's, in a home; our son had surgery; and our daughter had a skin cancer that needed to be removed (thank God for the positive outcomes for our children). These events plus all the other trials and tribulations of life—work, stress, moving, and relationships—are the complex tapestry of existence that make being alive worthwhile. We realized how vulnerable we all are to illness and disease, no matter where we are or in what phase of life we find ourselves.

Taking good care of oneself is critical to a full life. Listening to your body is vital to remaining healthy. Additionally, it helped us realize there are other people that need your love and attention during the healing process. The rest of your life does not simply shut down as you are living through the healing process; it is expanded in a new way. Now these experiences can be put into a new framework of existence. Life really does go through stages, and accepting this only makes it easier.

While we were struggling through the prostate cancer, the other experiences in our family let us know we all have challenges in life that we each deal with in our own way, and that the goal is to lead a happy and healthy life with a great deal of love. Ultimately, those struggles can have outcomes that range from death to being healthier than ever. These experiences in our family were examples for us to learn together. Tears of sadness, tears of laughter, tears of remembering, tears of healing—they all were meaningful and necessary, because as we entered into the Circle of Healing and went through it, all of life's other events continued to happen around us. We learned from them, stressed about them, and continued to live our lives through them.

Family members can play many roles while you are involved in the healing process. They can be listeners, organizers, researchers, appointment makers, lovers, supporters, and caregivers, whatever is required, depending on your individual needs and their individual capabilities, they are there for you. Cancer is frightening to family members, especially to partners and children.

They might wonder how the family patriarch could be physically weak and sick. It challenges core beliefs of the role of the father as leader of the family and invincible. It can be a very difficult time for all, and there is no right or wrong way for a family member to react. Any judgment about the situation should be set aside and replaced with thoughts of hope, faith, and love. Past relationships and feelings that have been buried can emerge and allow for healing for all. As time passes, relationships can change or they can remain the same; this is dependent on the dynamics of the family and its members.

Your family may or may not comprehend the scope of what is happening. Some might not be as concerned because they are not living with the experience day in and day out. They may be coping with their own issues, and it might be unreasonable to expect the relationship to be stronger and healthier than before the cancer. Your family is always your family, and through the good times and the bad times, through the moments of intense despair, they will still be your family. They are in your heart and mind even if they are not physically in your presence. They have been in your past, exist in your present, and can be an important part of your reason to heal and cure yourself. While you cannot change your past together, you can take each moment in the future as an opportunity to show them you love them and to reach out to them when you have the strength to give of yourself. As loving family members, they hopefully will understand that during the time you are fighting cancer, you may not be there for them as much as they might want, because you just don't have the energy to do more. It is a time when it is wise to pay silent tribute for what you have, preserve the energy you have to heal, and be grateful for the unconditional love of family if that is what you have. By being involved in this horrific and frightening experience, each family member can emerge with a higher sense of purpose to live a life of love, compassion, and forgiveness.

Questions they are probably asking themselves but are too afraid to discuss with you can be very frightening and upsetting for them. Here are some of the questions that might be on their minds:

- How can my husband (partner) and my love, be sick?
- What do you mean my dad (brother, uncle) has cancer?
- How can my older brother be dying?

- Why is this happening to my son—he's so young?
- Why didn't I spend more time with my dad?
- What did we do that caused my husband to get cancer?
- How can I tell him how afraid I am for him and for us?

These types of questions can open your mind to the possibility that the loved ones in your life are facing their own set of issues. Because of this, support from family can be complicated. Each family member is trying to cope with this issue in his or her own way, plus trying to be loving and caring for their father, brother, or partner who has cancer. What you learn is that each family member will cope with this on a very individual basis. Some will ask you right away how you're doing; others may never ask you. It all depends on how they are dealing with this issue themselves. Additionally, what the family members are hearing may be getting processed much differently than how you processed learning about your cancer.

There is an important dynamic going on if you are the prostate-cancer patient. You are the person who is ill and trying to focus on getting well and, concurrently, trying to protect his family. This may be the first time your family sees you as vulnerable, which could be a very uncomfortable role for you. All at once you are dealing with your mortality and, at the same time, perhaps feeling pressure or a desire to keep up with your role as the head of the household. Be prepared for this struggle because at times you may only be in the role of patient. If you are interacting with your family, you will probably want to make sure you are emotionally energized to play the role of family leader. This is especially relevant if you are into your treatment phase, recovering from surgery, or having radiation; at those times you will be very tired and might be experiencing pain from the recovery.

Family support is a two-way street. You will get support from your family as you simultaneously give them support. Most people think it goes only one way, from the healthy family member to the family member with cancer, but it does not. How do you deal with this? In most cases, this is one of the most difficult challenges of coping with the disease. There you are, struggling to heal, to be around for the next twenty to thirty years or even longer, and at the same time you are trying to continue as the family leader. It is not easy, and the past cannot be repeated. You have cancer, and you, as the family leader, are now vulnerable and could even die.

As a spouse or partner, you are trying to create a place where the miracle of healing can happen and to comfort and protect your loved one from all this pain and sadness. This can be exceedingly stressful on your relationship, even though both partners are trying their best.

In terms of your children (if you have any) and your immediate family, you may want them to be able to understand what is going on and at the same time not want them to worry. You may want to make them as happy as they can be, in spite of all your pain, fear, and concern. This can be very challenging, especially if your kids or immediate family do not live in the same community or general area, as in our case, because you may not be sure exactly how much you want to tell them or how much detail you want to go into. We found that telling them all the details was not necessary or meaningful. It might have been too much for all involved.

The energy you need to heal is grueling, and you need to be able to count on yourself to be dedicated to healing yourself. Those in the healing process are too busy healing, and those removed from the healing process have no sense of the full challenge. Quite frankly, the geographical distance can help one remain partially detached. It will allow other family members to provide their innocent and unfettered support, the unconditional love they want to provide to help the healing process. This option can be a way for all to cope with the situation and not add any more stress to the lives of all involved. Taking an approach like this can work to keep everyone with a contributing role without too much pain and suffering.

If you decide to go into all the details with family members, help them educate themselves about the disease. Encourage them to go to prostate-cancer-specific Web sites, information sources, libraries, and a variety of books that have been published on the subject. This will help all of you have a more productive discussion about your disease. They will be able to be less emotional and more objective about your condition.

Friends

Friends can play an important role in your life when you have cancer, because they can be more removed than your family. As a result, they have the ability to be more objective with you and can be a great way to escape conversations and thoughts about your cancer. Jim and I were lucky to have such a strong and encouraging network of friends. Simple things like dinners and social engagements were key to taking heavy issues off our minds for a while. Laughter and fun are critical to cope, and friends can deliver experiences filled with both.

Remember that as you are trying to understand the disease and what it means to you personally, the reality is your friends may not have the ability to cope with everything you are going through. The details of prostate cancer get quite involved and personal. You may want to consider how you will or will not discuss the disease with your friends. If the information you provide them is too complicated, they may not be capable of understanding what you are talking about. It is not that they don't want to, it is just that they have not been living through the experience like you have. They do not have the full view and can't interpret the experience and see it through your eyes. Additionally, they may not have the time to learn the details of what you are now exposed to.

While your friends care about you and love you, they may be filled with their own fear. In many cases, they may have limited knowledge of dealing with this form of cancer, especially if it is at a life-threatening stage. This can cause your relationship to get complicated and confusing. This may seem unfair. However, it is important to be aware that relationships with friends can change as a result of your illness—some for the better, some for the worse.

Conferences and Seminars

One critical point we learned from a seminar was how importantly support groups figured in long-term survival rates. This was an activity Jim would not have pursued willingly had he not heard for himself the power of support groups. We were right in the middle of Jim's healing process with radiation therapy and were eager to hear as much as we could about what other prostate-cancer sufferers were doing. We arranged to go to the first annual Prostate Cancer Conference, at the University of Michigan, in Ann Arbor, Michigan. The conference was attended by more than five hundred people and was an excellent opportunity to meet them and hear different stories about prostate cancer, treatments, and other issues.

During this conference, there was a fair amount of discussion about the clinical trials; and other information and sources came up as well. Informal newsletters, US TOO! International, CapCure, and a great deal more.

One presentation that had meaning for us was about the fact that one drug, Proscar, was found to be effective in only 5 percent of the patients when taken with Lupron and Casodex as a part of hormone therapy. As a result, the medical community was not recommending it as a generally accepted treatment. What? Were they crazy? What happened if you were in the 5 percent? How would you feel? We went back to our doctors and made sure Jim received that drug. When it has a personal impact on you personally and you are fighting this disease with all your energy, 5 percent—one out of twenty—seems like worthwhile odds to pursue.

Five Reasons To Attend at Least One Seminar

- Meet new people who you will talk to openly about prostate cancer.
- Become aware of resources and professionals that are available to you.
- Expose yourself to other points of view that are beyond your own and that of your doctors.
- Keep grounded in what is really important—your health.
- Have fun, because even though you have cancer, it doesn't mean you can't enjoy life or these types of events.

Support can manifest itself in many forms. One of the best ways to learn about what is going on in the treatment of prostate cancer is to attend prostate-cancer conferences and seminars. Often key conferences will have leading doctors and researchers discussing the most current learning in the field. The conferences usually run for two days and have speakers on all aspects of the disease, from the medical and physical side to the human and emotional side.

The costs for attendance ranges from free to a few hundred dollars plus travel expenses (if required). Here are two of the larger conferences to consider:

- University of Michigan Annual Prostate Cancer Symposium, in Ann Arbor—Usually held in the summer.
- US TOO! National Meeting—Usually held in the fall in a host city that changes annually.

Support Groups

After the information from the conference Jim signed up for a support group. Jim would go weekly to his support group and come home "worse" than when he left—sadder, more detached, and deeply upset—and as his partner I had to question why, why, why encourage and then let him go? This is part of the "going through" process of cancer as opposed to going around it. While I really was concerned about the support-group meetings because of how they affected Jim, I knew the results were well worth it. Support groups are a must for all, especially the person living with the disease and their significant partner.

It is interesting to realize those in the support group, who never knew your husband, your father, or your friend (and partner), might be the best support system. Why? Because they are there, in the same situation. They also have the disease, and they understand the fear. They are sad, too. They have the same feelings, the same symptoms, and the same side effects. They can totally understand what your loved one is going through. Jim happened to be the youngest and one of the most ill members in the group, with one of the highest PSAs.

How can I describe the transformation I would experience in Jim after support groups? Tears, tears, so many tears—not initially visible, they were bottled up inside. It was only when I would probe him as to why he was upset, and visibly tense, and push for him to share, that the tears would flow—a small trickle from the corner of his eyes and then, once released, like a rivulet running down a mountain, a stream of tears for himself, for his support group, for the unknown, and for the known.

There are no excuses necessary in support groups. How weird and how wonderful—a place where you can just be. The group was a place where things—sometimes quiet and sometimes sad and sometimes totally misunderstood were happening. It was tragic and magic at the same time.

Jim's support group was part of a study that was being observed by UCSF. There were two members of the UCSF staff at most meetings taking notes and listening. On occasion they would interact, but they were really there just to observe. There were twelve people in the group from all demographic and ethnic backgrounds. This added greatly to the experience, because they had such diverse points of view.

Usually one of the UCSF doctors would kick off the meeting by saying, "Does anybody want to start us off tonight?" Sure enough, one of the attendees would begin to talk about a topic that was on his mind. No subjects were off-limits; there were discussions about impotence, diapers, bleeding, fear of death, relationship management, and life in general. Each person had his own struggles and experiences to share, and the conversations flowed freely. The group met for ten weeks, and when it was over the participants decided that it was not enough for them. After a short break, they started sessions again for another round. The meetings were always on Tuesday nights, at the same time and place. This made it easy to remember, and they did not interfere with the weekend.

At one point, Jim and the other members learned that one of the members had developed a cancerous brain tumor. This was profoundly difficult, because each week Jim would see the slow death of a support-group partner. Two months after the meetings ended, we called him to drop off a holiday gift, only to get voice mail. Prior to leaving town for the Christmas holiday, we dropped off the gift at his door—again to no answer. In our hearts we suspected that life may have been coming to an end. We returned after the first of the year and we learned, much to our sadness, that our fears were justified and Jim's friend had died. We sat on our couch and cried, feeling free to do so without judging each other, but with the reassurance to love each other fully each day. It is tragic and sad to lose someone and realize that you, too, may die the same way. The reality of it is almost too much to cope with. How can I explain the power of tears? They heal, they humble us, and they show we care. They let us grow through our innermost feelings. When we shed tears, it is like a dam releasing an emotional flood.

The Role of the Spouse or Partner

The role of the partner of a cancer patient is one of unending giving, but what you get in return is unending appreciation, gratitude, and love. As the partner, you have the chance to have a real purpose in life, to love another more deeply than you ever dreamed possible, to rise to the occasion and share all the wonderful talents you have been given to help your partner "in sickness and in health." The emotional dam keeps rising and we become swollen inside until, like a storm-filled dam, we eventually overflow. At first, there is an initial tear or two as we try to hold the feelings back, but eventually we are overcome with emotion. There is a bursting of the unstoppable, overwhelming sadness that created those rivers of tears. Those streams of tears connect the sadness in one's soul with the body. (Accept them as a power of connection rather than being opposed to denial and repression.) Tears heal. The deepness by which you learn to live your life can be forever changed in a way that brings a richness of joy and pleasure, because you have given yourself freely to another.

Often, I found myself making sure I would try to be positive about events even if they seemed terrible. Most likely my background in marketing made me "spin" even the events in our own lives. This made reality easier to swallow because what I perceived was a rose-colored version of it. Personally, this worked for me as it has for all of my adult life. My favorite tactic when things are seriously wrong is to convince others and myself that "it will be fine." The worse the situation, the more frequently I utter this expression as my coping mechanism. It lets me stay in the moment without letting my mind race with negativity. Even though negative thoughts would still manifest themselves, I was able to get by with a positive outlook, and hope that things actually would be fine. The space where I believed that "it will be fine" suited me perfectly.

While you are not the person with cancer, you have your own internal struggles that can seem insurmountable at times. Fearing what your life and the life of your children will be like without your partner is the worst worry, and the consequent lack of sleep this may bring can run you down. But being strong and optimistic is vital. Being the ultimate cheerleader and a pillar of strength is tough when you are frightened and depressed, but you do it. You do it because you love him. You cry to family and friends or at support groups; you get help. You take care of yourself. You go through the motions. You get through it. You remember that prostate cancer has a high survival rate and that the odds are in your favor. You survive, and give him the strength to do the same. As Lao-TZE said, "Because of deep love, we are courageous."

Using this time to get involved in alternative healing arts can be a healthy and interesting diversion. Try acupuncture.

Go to yoga. Get a massage. Develop your own regime of herbs, vitamins, and minerals. Become a healthy cook. Bring health and light and life to your home. And remember that there are other women and male partners going through the same thing. Find them!

Books such as *Love and Survival* by Dr. Dean Ornish and *Emotional Intelligence* by Daniel Goleman are must-reads for partners. Goleman explains the biological ramifications of our emotions and the importance of letting go of the emotions like anger and fear for better health. In his book, Dr. Ornish deals with issues of love and intimacy and both the healing and illness causing powers that they can create. We learn that our nurturing love can have an enormous impact on healing those we love.

Seeking spirituality for myself and to accept life's mysteries has given me great peace, especially during Jim's cancer. Books like *How to Know God* by Deepak Chopra and *Illuminata* by Marianne Williamson are invaluable resources to keep partners grounded in faith and help us learn to overcome pain with prayer.

Voices of Healing

When most people think of support groups, they usually don't think of a mixed, eclectic group of all types of folks with all types of diseases. California's progressive social nature is very conducive to support groups like Voices of Healing. It is run in and around the Bay Area and offers people a place to share their feelings about their experiences with illness and pain. A man I had worked with at Pepsico had referred Jim and me to this group.

Initially, we were too busy with other treatments and getting through the cancer experience to add this, but we opted to try it one night. The meeting was held at Fort Mason by the Marina, in San Francisco, and it was free unless you wanted to make a donation. There were ten people at the meeting—one other couple, a therapist facilitator, three other women, and two men. Many of the attendees had chronic diseases, including persistent back pain, ovarian cancer, and multiple sclerosis. Many distressed people—it was another sad moment. How did I miss all these people before this? Suddenly, I was much more aware of how many people in the world live with pain and suffering every day and had for years.

Both Jim and I sat, listened, and absorbed it all. Tales of doctors not believing that the person really was in pain and refusing to treat it, and of being misdiagnosed. Sitting there, I felt lucky we had not experienced these horrible types of events. There was a point in the meeting when each person had to talk about what change the disease had caused in their lives. Jim spoke about his ability to live in the present as opposed to the past or the future. My comments surprised me because I said that the disease had shown me much of what we do is really unimportant. The disease enables and forces Jim and me to spend more time together. We were joined together fighting cancer, and this had become our raison d'etre. As I said, "I am not glad Jim has cancer, but I am grateful for the time we spend together in life now more than ever before." Tears welled up in my eyes, and my voice started to crack. The others in the room understood what I meant. Time had taken on a special new meaning in all of our lives. Jim placed his arm around me and kissed my forehead, a beautiful gesture, and then it was the next person's turn to speak.

Some prostate-cancer patients and their families do not appreciate the intrinsic value of support groups. Too many support groups sound anemic, weak, but in reality that is far from true. They are filled with people who are not bystanders but in the trenches. Members of a support group are on a level playing field playing against prostate cancer and playing to win. They, too, are struggling with the details of their disease, and they truly understand what it is to live through this kind of experience. The members of the groups are all ill, and they are usually highly committed to sharing their experiences and to live through them to the best of their ability. Support groups are not just a group of grumpy old men getting together to bitch and moan. It is an opportunity to share the thoughts that you can't say to your wife, your best friend, or your doctor—those deep-down thoughts that only you know you have.

Support-group sessions can be very intense. It is such a time of openness, a time for men to discuss their fears through man-to-man sharing. Each man with his own experiences, challenges, and potential of death—the conversations can be emotionally overwhelming, but they are vital. They allow each member to release all their negative energy and fears in a place where there is no judging one another. There are also support groups for cancer survivors, couples, and continuing wellness. Check with your hospital, house of worship, or community health service, which should be able to provide you with a number of options depending on your needs.

Your Network

- **Family and Friends:** Whom else can you reach out to during this time? Have you practiced alone how to tell your family and friends before you actually share the news? Do you know others who have gone through cancer? What other resources do you have to draw on to give you strength during this time? How actively do you want to engage your family in your treatment? How much do you want to share with your partner or other family members? How do you want to tell them? Will you see them during treatment?
- **Bring it all together:** Have you thought about how you will bring all the wonderful resources together that you have available? Do you want to write down a plan? Do you intend to be informal and let events unfold as they may?
- **Support:** Do you plan on attending support groups? Alone? With your spouse or significant other? Where are the support groups in your town—at the hospital, at your house of worship, or elsewhere?
- **Mental:** How are you feeling? Are you removed from your family and friends? Are you depressed? Should you ask the doctor for an antidepressant or some other alternative? Have you cried yet? How often are you crying? (If daily, please tell your doctor; other than that you're probably just fine.) Are you losing your temper or having great mood swings often? Are you drinking more? Watch these signs for depression.
- **Spirituality:** Do you go to church, temple, or other place of worship? Do you plan to get involved in any form of spiritual practice? Have you meditated on cancer or talked to God about cancer? Are you comfortable with your relationship with your spiritual self? Do you have or even want one? Would you consider other ways you can add to your spiritual life, such as reading inspirational books and articles, attending seminars, or going on a retreat?

Certainly these are not all the questions you will want to ask yourself. They are a great starting point for entering the implementation phase of the Circle of Healing.

PART THREE
LIVING WITH CANCER

LIFE IN THE CANCER YEARS

I know God won't give me anything I can't handle; I just wish he wouldn't trust me so much.

—Mother Teresa

The following few pages will give you a glimpse of some of our highs and lows as we implemented the healing action plan. Hopefully you will get the sense that it is possible to emerge as a stronger, healthier human being—more fulfilled in life and with an appreciation of being alive.

Breast Cancer, Too?

Now it was my turn to go through the fear and panic of cancer. This was not good, a note from a doctor after my mammogram: "We need you to come back in based on the initial results of your mammogram. We need to take a second look." This happened not just once but twice during Jim's treatment.

The first time it was in January, four months after Jim had completed radiation. My parents were visiting the day the letter arrived. I felt awful, afraid, replaying the scenes in my mind from our experience with Jim, remembering this as exactly the way it started—one small test, one small unusual result, one small communication from the doctor and our entire world was sent into a tailspin. Could this be happening again? I did not have the heart to tell anyone, not Jim, my parents, no one. That night I was not able to sleep. It was strange, but I was thinking maybe if it was cancer, Jim and I would be even closer. Then I truly would be experiencing cancer like him—as a victim, as an individual trying to beat the disease, angry at my body and fearful for my life. The next day I went into the bedroom and discreetly made an appointment to go back to the facility and have my breast reexamined. I didn't want to go. I didn't want to have to deal with the outcome if it was negative. I was afraid and wondered how much more we could take.

Thinking again on the drive to the office, "If I have cancer, if this is the case, I will handle it. I will be able to experience the same feelings as Jim. If he could get through this, so can I." I realized by my reaction how much guilt I felt about Jim having cancer and my being healthy. Never before had this feeling bubbled up from my inner thoughts. Like an unending mountain spring, new feelings seem to constantly emerge with cancer. For some reason, one's senses feel heightened, and the emotions are much deeper, fuller, and rawer than before. Maybe it keeps one on the edge—always ready to jump.

Luckily, the breast-cancer scare turned out to be nothing but one more bump in the road. A physical with no follow-up and nothing to do sounded ideal and was the result after the big scare.

Jim's Dream

After radiation, Jim continued to be dedicated to the healing process. Supposedly it is common to have vivid dreams when suffering from cancer, and he had a few fitful nights after the first weeks. He would bolt awake during the night, his mind screaming with angst, the perpetual nightmare of fear and panic when one is faced with his mortality, the lack of control over the future and life-and-death decisions. This was only natural—his mind was racing with all those choices. What is the best thing to do? How do you know if the doctors don't know?

One night, almost as a call from his subconscious to calm and reassure his conscious mind, he dreamed, "I am healed." The signal was so strong, it shot through his body like an electric shock; the message so powerful, he instantly woke from a sound sleep. He had the dream only once. We were both ecstatic the next morning when Jim shared the experience, because he didn't usually remember his dreams. We celebrated at breakfast by taking precious time to bask together in the reassuring feeling. For a few hours that morning we read the daily papers, appreciating those moments without fear and filled with hope. We genuinely believed this was a sign of Jim's survival, and, as eternal optimists, we accepted that Edgar Allan Poe was right when he wrote, "All that we see or seem is but a dream within a dream."

An Alarming Phone Call

Good results from tests and PSA counts are like good grades from college if you are trying to get into a top grad school—they mean everything. After twelve months, Jim went for his normal PSA checkup and was feeling great until he received one short, sixty-second phone call that night. We were sitting at our dining room table recapping the day, when the phone rang. Normally we try not to pick up the phone during our conversations, but we were waiting for what we thought were sure to be good test results. Jim picked up the receiver. On the other end of the line was the nurse from UCSF. She was calling to give Jim the results, as she had during the last nine months.

The nurse was brief, telling Jim his PSA was below .2. There was a look of absolute panic on Jim's face. He numbly acknowledged the information and hung up the phone. Jim's last test had been below .02 (considered "undetectable" by the doctors, meaning no sign of cancer cells.) A test score of .2 meant that the cancer had multiplied ten times since the last test, less than 90 days. This news was in the details, details that added up to the devastating possibility of a reemergence of cancer.

Both of us went off the deep end with immediate thoughts of despair, sadness, and sheer panic. Could this really be happening? What would we do now? How fast was the cancer growing? Everything seemed to be going so well, hadn't it? How would we deal with this new situation; how would our life change again?

Our minds were racing with concern for the future, because by then we had learned that from test results like this, the doctor can fairly accurately predict how fast the cancer is growing and how much time it will take for the cancer to be a serious problem again. In this case, the preliminary data from the test seemed to indicate Jim's cancer was growing very fast again and the outcome could be the early end of Jim's life.

As we sat at dinner, neither of us was hungry anymore. That night Jim and I were unusually quiet—like a night in the backwoods, quiet and in shock. What could we say? We thought we were on the right track, and now this. No symptoms, no grand announcement, just one little number, one *very* small number that could change our world. As Jim told me, he had burst into tears. Both of us were thinking to ourselves, Why? What would we do?

First I brought up the fact that during our discussions with the doctors they had told us that until the score went over 2 the long-term prognosis could still be good. Maybe this would be okay even though it was not what we wanted to hear. The idea that the cancer may be growing again caused us great fear. It was a sleepless night: We hugged each other and tossed and turned, and arose at four. We decided in the morning to call back to get more details from the nurse. We asked about the test results and our next steps.

Unbelievably, we found out that the test was a different one than the previous PSA tests Jim had taken. Yes, it still measured PSA, but it did not measure PSA to lower levels. This was fantastic news. Jim did not have a problem; the cancer was still contained. We were still okay; Jim was still on the road to healing and curing in spite of the call.

Jim asked the nurse why he was given a different test. What we learned was that the insurance company did not want to pay for the more expensive PSA test that measured to the sensitivity of .02 and below, but would only authorize tests that measured to .2 and below. Believe me, now we definitely ask which type of PSA test we are taking.

My Back Is Killing Me!

By now we had lived with cancer for over fifteen months and were feeling that Jim was on the road to a full recovery. After we had been through all the shots, the months of radiation, the herbs, the trainer, the acupuncturist, the daily drugs, and the meditation, we thought the rest would all go smoothly. Surprise! Even with excellent planning life doesn't always unfold as we expect. After the supposedly successful and aggressive radiation and approximately one year after diagnosis, Jim started to have ongoing backaches. The backaches were influencing his ability to move freely and sleep without waking up during the evening. As we knew from reading about advanced stages of prostate cancer, metastatic prostate cancer in most cases spreads to one's lungs and bones. We also knew there was evidence that radiation and other treatments can mask the spread of the cancer.

Jim thought his back pain might be serious because it was constant and nagging. Honestly, I have to say at that point I had no fortitude left to handle more angst or emotional pain associated with disease. It was defeating me, little by little wearing me down. Perseverance was required for this battle, so I mustered up all my forces. I was not going to cater to this sensation, and I would not give in because my husband's life was at stake; our life together was at stake. We just had to lift ourselves up and keep being a positive force, one with the hope and belief that it really could be okay in spite of the terror we were facing.

Initially, I tried to convince Jim the pain was from our daily running or perhaps a by-product of a day when he had slept on a less-than-perfect hotel bed. I didn't want to even consider another reason and truly wouldn't be able to cope with any other. Hadn't we been through enough?

But the pain persisted, and we knew Jim had to address it with his doctor. At our next doctor's visit, which took place less than two weeks later, we brought it up. The doctor, too, hoped it could be running-related, and he proscribed Jim a powerful pain reliever to relieve the discomfort. But the pain continued, so we convinced the doctor to explore other potential causes. The doctor scheduled the required tests, including a bone-densitometry test and a complete set of back X-rays. Without Jim's speaking up, none of this would have happened. When you have pains or unusual side effects, speak up. Otherwise, you may actually be hurting your chances for recovery. Put the macho-man thing behind you and listen to your body. If you are in pain, there is something wrong and painkillers only dull the senses, they do not solve the root cause of the problem.

The bone-densitometry test showed a loss of bone mass, a precursor to the beginning of osteoporosis, which was a potential side effect of all the drugs—and nothing to mess around with. However, this test does not tell you the cause, and though we now knew we had a problem, the reason was uncertain. Jim had been lifting weights and exercising, and we felt scared because healthy bones should have been the benefit of his hard work. Could the cancer have been in his bones already? We already knew the cancer was highly likely to be metastatic. Could it have settled in one of its favorite places, the bones of the lower back and pelvis? Terrible thoughts, and Jim was in pain. We scheduled the X-rays for the following week. That weekend was rough:

tears, concern, uncertainty, just like when we had first started. But now we had more data and knew that this could be bad, very bad. Jim went for X-rays, and I joined him.

More tests, new procedures—again we accepted them but, at the same time, hated to see them. Watching Jim, making sure he was checked in properly, getting him water, making sure he was called in for his tests before too long. The X-rays were standard back X-rays, but they were terrifying for us. The outcome was unknown, and we had already been through so much. They x-rayed him from all sides—front, back, and both sides—a simple procedure. The technician developed the slides; a "hot spot" was visible on several of them. This looked very bad indeed. I was standing behind the technician and saw the mounted X-rays. Without any medical training, I could even see a bright spot. Could this be cancer in his back? Fear overwhelmed me, scared me to death. There was a bright, light section at the base of Jim's spine. It did not look like the rest of his back X-ray. Trying to keep calm as I asked the technician what it could be. "Well," he said, "I can't tell you anything. You will have to get a diagnosis from the doctor. He will call you early next week."

Friday we called the doctor, and got no return call. Another awful weekend. On Monday morning we called again. The doctor told us that Jim had lower back degeneration, but that the cause was unknown. Mercifully, it was definitely not cancer but was the cause of the pain he was experiencing. With this new information, we elatedly went back to our radial oncologist for treatment. Ironic—now the situation seemed tolerable because it was not from the Big "C", cancer. He prescribed Fosomax and painkillers. Jim takes Fosomax daily to strengthen his bones. Fosomax is a very strange drug. It must be taken in the morning on an empty stomach, but you cannot stay in bed because it makes you feel like you are choking. As far as the painkillers go, Jim has taken about ten in two years. One more hurdle, one more sign. It's true: "What doesn't kill me makes me stronger." Still, the feeling that this cancer may never be over is always there, lurking cruelly.

Yet Another Scare

While the initial treatment from the radiation went well, about one year afterward Jim continued to have rectal bleeding.

Ideally, this should have ceased after radiation, but it had not. There was enough concern from his radial oncologist about colon cancer or other major complications that, rather than be uncertain, our doctors recommended we go to a colon/lower gastrointestinal specialist.

Between the doctors' visits and the trip to the specialist, we both experienced an eerie feeling. We had already been through enough—the emotions of Jim having cancer, then the treatments, then the hopeful feeling that had weathered the storm. Now, here we were again—with uncertainty and fear. It was unbelievably upsetting. Jim was really worried about this. He tried to pass it off as just another task we had to deal with, put on our calendars, and schedule—and it would be over, right? Maybe. The anticipation and anxiety were straining us. I was not able to sleep at night. Jim was able to sleep without a hitch—undoubtedly a combination of the drugs and his body's healing. I spun in a downward cycle. The more anxiety built with me, the harder it was to sleep. The more tired I became, the more worried, the less I slept. It was awful, and yet we didn't talk about it with anyone. We didn't want to have anyone worrying, knowing, or asking us at such a low, dark period for us. When you have a sense even though you wish, pray, think, believe it will be okay, that there is still the chance of a problem, how does one cope? How could Jim cope with this? It would be too hard for us. I couldn't share these fears with Jim; he needed me to be there for him, the optimistic side reinforcing what we wished to be true. Yet my fear was ever present: what would it be like if this was colon cancer? What if he would die and he wouldn't be in my life? Overwhelmed the first time, I tried to cope. The fear of cancer a second time was almost too much to bear. But despite my intense sadness and anxiety, I continued to do what I always do as a coping mechanism: I worked out, I worked, and I became ultra, ultra busy. This caused Jim and me to talk a little less, enabling us to survive this dark period.

We went to the hospital, and Jim was prepped to go into the operating room. The doctor came in, much more comfortable with the process than we and ready to go. He had a schedule. To him this was just part of his day; to us this was one of those big life days, when what happens can change everything. His manner was professional as he described vividly the process Jim would be going through. I felt sick when I heard it, but I knew Jim was watching for my visible cues, my mental reinforcement. It will be fine! I tried my best to keep my face still. It doesn't sound too bad, does it? But I was thinking, Oh, my God, this is awful. Is he going to be okay through this? After all, he is bleeding down there, could it be complications? But there I stood holding his hand, with the doctor, nurse, and the ultrasound machine beside us.

The doctor told us the procedure would last about an hour unless there were complications or he needed to do additional exploratory actions. There would be a waiting room for me down the hall. I would just wait—and he would let me know the outcome after the procedure was complete. We counted with Jim as the anesthesia drugs quickly took over. We counted together, ten, nine . . . by eight he was out like a light. I left him to the uncertainty, grateful I was able to stay with him right to his last moment of consciousness.

I left the operating room and, feeling overwhelmed, started to cry. What would I do? What if; what if? I made it to the waiting room, and was there all alone with no TV or current magazines to distract me. As was our usual procedure, we had tried to get Jim scheduled as the first appointment of the day. No reasons to pine away all day, plus doctors don't control their own schedules and can get easily delayed. After about twenty minutes I walked down to Jim's recovery room. They didn't want me to wait there because patients would be comong in to undress. I wanted to make sure the hangers they promised for Jim's trousers and jacket were there. They were there, and I hung up his clothes, placing them with care and attention in the narrow closet. As I was doing this I stopped, grabbed the jacket to my face, and smelled it. It smelled of Jim. How I loved him! Even such an object, just a thing, was redolent of him. I knew the smell. It made me feel warm and safe, aligned with Jim and happy while I was in such a dreary place at such an uncertain and scary time. In a strange sort of way, I felt happy—his smell, there to comfort me. I left the room. I wanted his smell to stay with me forever, like a lucky charm around my neck to know all was well, no matter what.

Finally, the doctor came out to find me. Jim was through the surgery and had been brought to the recovery area. The doctor was there to let me know how it had gone, touching me on the shoulder. I knew without words, without even seeing him, that it was okay, my Jim was okay. An overwhelming sense of relief overcame me to the core of my soul. Inside, an amazing sense of—relief . . . thank you, thank you! Breathing out a big sigh, releasing the fear, all the worry, and the sadness. This seemed to happen in a nanosecond, because as the doctor's eyes connected with mine, he said, "Mrs. Miller, I want you to know Jim is just fine." That was enough for me. No more details, I just wanted to know where he was, when could I see him. The other details seemed unimportant then. No cancer—that was all I cared about then.

It had been a full day and it wasn't even ten in the morning. I sat there for about an hour and was grateful, numb and oblivious to the passage of time. After another hour the nurse came to get me. Jim seemed to be partially awake but was still very drowsy. I could go to the recovery room and sit with him and help him get up, take in liquids, and start to get reoriented to where he was.

When I went to see Jim, I could tell he still was out of it, totally drugged up, but his first few words captured it all. "Do I have cancer?" No matter the drugs, surgery, lack of rest, it was there strongly, the subconscious fear and awareness of what was going on today. He wanted to know. All I said was, "You are great, and the doctor said there is no cancer." As the last syllable left my lips, he fell back to sleep. With an ever-so-small smile on his face he drifted off for over two hours, a clear indication he was utterly exhausted by this experience. When you are not living it, it is hard to explain, but our fear of the cancer had returned absolutely devastated both of us.

Holiday Blues

The holidays are notorious for adding stress and strain to peoples' lives. Never before had this affected us the way it did the first Christmas after Jim was diagnosed with prostate cancer. We were hesitant to go out to many events because Jim was feeling tired from the drugs and probably mildly depression. We were going through all the motions of festivities and fun, but, on the inside, we were both dreading many of the days.

Christmas was always Jim's favorite time of year because of his retail background, gifts and giving and the excitement of the season. Having spent the previous twenty-plus years as a retail executive, he was experiencing the Christmas season without the same sense of the holidays. This manifested itself in ways, like not wanting to send cards to communicate what was happening to us. The holidays seemed to be a time to spread happy news and good cheer, not news of cancer. While we were doing as well as we could do with Jim's PSA at .02 undetectable, we felt it was premature to share this information with others. Additionally, based on the last ten months, neither of us really had the energy to do more than make it through the season and be thankful for the last year of detection and initial treatments. We were exhausted.

Our friends were terrific to us during this time, inviting us to parties and events. We tried to attend most of them and managed this by arriving early and leaving before 10:00 P.M. Jim did not have the strength or stamina for more. Often with restaurant reservations, we would suggest meeting at 6:00 P.M. and having an early dinner. While hardly noticeable to our friends, it was a way we could get Jim home by 9:30 or 10:00. His body needed the rest, and he would literally pass out from exhaustion. All the treatments, drugs, and healing of his body depleted his energy by the end of the day.

One evening we went out to dinner at a dear friend's place in Alamo, a suburb of San Francisco. Our friends, the Gavigans, always had a special dinner party during the holidays. The evening was lovely. At one point, we were all chatting as we retired to the family room to be by the crackling fireplace and beautiful-smelling fir tree. Out of nowhere, our situation hit me like a ton of bricks. One of our friends asked me about what was happening with Jim, but I had to keep my feelings inside and always try to be strong and positive. The combination of the holidays, being with friends, and the realization that next year might be very different made me want to stop the world right there, and have time stand still so Jim could be with us next year and all the years after that without any concern. It was too much for me, and I broke into tears. Fortunately, only the host and one other guest were there at the moment. I felt terrible about what happened, but it was out of my control. Those feelings were intense; they cut me open like a knife and a wound of sadness bled from my heart. It was as if the ache in my heart had to be released from my body to enable me to accept what was.

Luckily, I gained my composure after a few minutes and went into the powder room. There I held a cold washcloth to my eyes to keep them from getting puffy. I emerged, released but tender. I was ready to make it through the rest of the holiday season without breaking down, but that proved to be impossible. At certain times, especially toward the end of the day, sadness would overwhelm me. The joy of the holidays matched with the fear of the disease made tears appear without warning. Tears became a means for me to release my emotions—happy or sad, fearful or glad.

Radiation, Tattoos, and the Crystal

One of the things we learned from Jim's cancer was we were doing a lot more laughing and crying. We were more emotionally sensitive because of the illness. We decided that we would go together to the hospital for his preradiation-treatment appointment. By now, we had learned that being with each other during each phase of this was important to both of us. The UCSF hospital sits high on a hill in San Francisco, the Pacific Ocean just a couple of miles away. A constant, moist wind off the ocean whips around the hospital and research complex. It was at least five–ten degrees cooler on average than where we live in the city of San Francisco.

In a short sleeve shirt, not prepared for the cold rush of air exiting the car, I was stirred to attention by a blast of reality making me feel uncomfortable and chilly. Somehow this was appropriate, because inside my body, every time we went to a hospital a bone chilling feeling overwhelmed me. Externally, both Jim and I were eager about going to UCSF, because we felt we were putting into action a critical part of curing him. The radiation treatment was finally going to happen after five months of being on hormone therapy, acupuncture, herbs, and vitamins. This was an important milestone for us; because Jim's tumor had shrunk dramatically. Fortunately, this was exactly the outcome the doctors had been hoping for Jim.

As a research hospital, the facilities at UCSF are not the priority. The majority of funds are spent on doctors research and clinical trials. The radial oncology department was no exception. As we entered the hospital, we saw a sign for the department that led us toward steps to the basement. This seemed a metaphor for how low we were feeling. We were about as low as we could go in the hospital. There was no way to go but up and we were ready.

Our initial impression was of a waiting room filled with patients of all ages, nationalities, and stages of cancer. Our saddest moment was seeing a boy about seven or eight who had lost his hair and was thin as a rail, but still fighting for his life. His mother was there with him, and you could sense the worry she had for him. It put in perspective how fortunate we were that it was not our kids we were here with and, in a strange sort of way, that was comforting to us. It is terrible to have cancer, but the idea of your child having it was more unbearable than what we were experiencing.

As we approached the registration area, we were presented with a number of forms. Jim glanced down and saw his file. His chart was all ready to go, or so we thought initially. The only problem was that the file was for a Jim Miller born in the 1920s. Here we were, getting ready to start radiation therapy and thinking, Wow, if they can get that wrong, what else can happen? Rather than get all bent out of shape, we decided it was funny. After all, Jim was not eighty years old, and he certainly did not look like a man in his eighties—"At least not yet," Jim said, and we laughed. There, at the reception desk, our laughter helped diffuse the situation and get everyone through that awkward moment. The doctors were always very supportive of my being there, and when Jim went in for his radiation fitting, I stayed right with him.

Jim went off to change into a hospital gown to prepare for his next step. We had been told they were going to show him where he would be getting treated plus make molds of his legs. When Jim was changed, he went off to a patient's treatment room, and they placed me in a small lounge that was empty of life and energy. It was not fancy, but it was quiet. A quiet space—my anxiety level was rising, especially with so many sick people in the main waiting room.

Within a few minutes, they came for me and we were led into the area of the hospital where the radiation rooms and equipment were located. I watched as they made an impression of Jim's legs to hold them perfectly in line for the radiation. Having me there reassuring Jim and myself ("It will be fine!") took a lot of the anxiety out of the radiation experiences. We would talk right until the procedures started; this gave him very little time to get anxious, be alone, or feel isolated.

Because of the nature of 3-D radiation treatment, the body needs to be perfectly aligned with the intended application of the radiation beams. To assist the doctors to hit their mark consistently in each treatment, they opted to use tattoos—small pinpoint-size dots as markers for the initial beam setup. You can imagine the looks we get at parties when friends are discussing their kids or grandkids getting tattoos, and I say, "Oh, yes, Jim has tattoos, too." We had lots of fun teasing people, because he is such a conservative type of guy, not a typical tattoo person. Having some fun with the steps along the process really helps.

Another example of this was when he would get his shot and go see the acupuncturist on the same day. I'd call him "Pokey." What could he say? He had usually been pricked twenty to twenty-five times during these days, and it was a way for me to acknowledge what was happening to him without being down about it. A little humor and laughter goes a long way.

Much has been speculated about the benefits of crystals, and, while we know nothing about them, Jim was given a crystal by Peggy, the acupuncturist, to use in radiation therapy. We felt it was important to use this gift as a symbolic gesture toward the mental healing process—a kind of "special charm" to help him. The crystal was small, about two inches long, clear and white with no elaborate markings on it. Just a plain crystal, but what it did for Jim had true meaning.

Each day as he went to radiation, he took the crystal from the dashboard of the car and placed it in his pants pocket. For over three months, as he went into the radiation room and changed into his gown, he took the crystal out of his pant's pocket, placed it in his right hand and kept it there during treatment. The powerful healing had started; he aligned his body, mind, and soul in order to receive radiation and heal.

Each day he would hold that crystal in his right hand and pray to God: Thank you for letting me be here; thank you for letting me be healed and cured. Most of us would have been dreading this, and yet Jim's approach was the exact opposite—thank you, I appreciate being here so I may be healed. While there is no scientific evidence about this type of approach, he believes it was crucial to his success. He was accepting what he could not change, opening himself up to the treatments, and feeling grateful for the outcome.

While the crystal was tiny, it helped us pass the drudgery of the treatment to a cathartic part of the process. If the crystal was okay, Jim would be okay, too.

For those who get radiation, you'll discover that there is a slight charred smell exuded by a person undergoing treatment.

At first it is subtle, almost like a dull smoky scent. Almost like after a party when a few people have smoked cigarettes. As the radiation treatment progresses, the smell becomes stronger. When you kiss the patient, you can actually taste the smell of burning on their breath. It is ever so subtle, but it is unmistakable.

By the time Jim's treatment was over, the smell permeated his clothes, his body, and our bed. I didn't mention it to him. It seemed trite in relation to what we were going through, but it was very upsetting. You could actually smell the effect of the radiation burning his body on the inside. Was this treatment or some cruel punishment? I wondered with tears in my eyes. In reflection, the cancer was so severe that the radiation had to be powerful, and radiation bashing cancer cells with intense energy burns and kills them, and the by-product is a strange smell, a strange kiss, and strange sweat. If this happens to you, don't be surprised. Just remember, it is all part of the process.

The burning smell passed after the radiation treatment was over. Within eight months the smell left Jim and our home. Slowly, but with each day, his body healed and the smell left. Reflecting on this, it's interesting to consider the acupuncture principle about smell being an important indicator of what is happening in your body.

Making New Choices

With all that was going on, Jim realized he needed to stop and contemplate what he could do for himself during this time. He was going to need to remain on treatment longer that we initially thought, so he decided to use this as an opportunity to do what he wanted to do in life. It turned out Jim had always wanted to go get his doctorate but it was never the right time. He was too busy working to support the family to be able to take such a significant amount of time out for himself. Those were the right choices as the children were growing up, but now they were adults in their twenties. This was a time when Jim could take on a major initiative that was meaningful to him. He decided to explore getting an advanced degree.

After about two months of extensive research, he found that George Washington University, in Washington, D.C., offered the type of executive doctoral program he wanted. Jim is a big believer in leadership and adult learning and wanted to pursue this path. With the help of business colleagues, who wrote letters of recommendation, and his good test scores, he was able to get into the program. At first, it seemed like a bit much, but as Jim went to D.C. for four days every month, he was able to grow as a person and participate in a positive, major life experience. The classes started one year after we moved to San Francisco and continued for almost three years. Today, he is in the dissertation phase and a candidate for a doctorate degree.

SEX AND PROSTATE CANCER

Do not weep; do not wax indignant. Understand.

—Baruch Spinoza

In Jim's case, Lupron, Casodex, and Proscar blocked testosterone production; therefore, within two weeks of his treatments with the drugs, he began to lose his ability to get an erection. Prior to this time, we had an active sex life and enjoyed the physical and mental release that comes with sexual pleasure. With the sudden change in Jim's ability and desire to have sex, the result was much harder for me as the partner, because I still had my hormones and was as attracted to Jim as ever. We talked this over, but there was not much for us to do because the idea of sexual aids did not appeal to us and we thought Jim would be on hormone therapy for less than twelve months.

To curb my own sexual desire for Jim, I replaced it with other activities that gave me the feeling of intimacy. Jim and I would make sure we hugged and kissed throughout the day. There was still physical activity, and I enjoyed the attention. The reality was, as Jim's partner, his health and well-being surpassed my need for sex. Because of all the stress and anxiety surrounding our situation, my desire for sex decreased as well. It just did not seem as important right then.

As time passed, I was glad to hear news of a new drug for erectile dysfunction. Once Viagra was announced, we asked about it during our next doctor visit. The doctor thought it would work, and it did work well for Jim. We were back to being able to have sex, but Jim's passion was not there due to the lack of hormones. For the first year, we had no ability to have regular intercourse. Both Jim and I were united on this point. Time without sex was a small sacrifice for us to be able to spend the rest of our lives together.

Certainly, as his partner, it was not as easy for me to deal with, but Jim was very willing to participate in other intimate activities such as massage, exercising and kissing. While his experience did not generate any sexual energy, there was still affection, passion, love, and intimacy. It may be hard to understand, but this actually made us closer—without sex we learned more about being intimate with each other. Sharing our feelings and emotions and being able to share each other really put us in touch with who each other was as a person and a partner.

For most men, whether short or long-term, their sexual function is impeded, eliminated, or temporarily unavailable while engaged in treatment. This often rocks the very foundation of a man's opinion of himself and his masculinity. The potential impact on his sex life is one of the most difficult parts of prostate cancer. It is virtually unavoidable. Not only is he at risk of dying from the disease, but he is also probably going to lose his ability to perform sexually. The actual prognosis depends on his age, the success of surgery, and his body's ability to again produce testosterone after hormone therapy. Well, good news—sex does not equal love, and intimacy is still possible without a male orgasm or an ejaculation. Many times, orgasm will be possible, but there will be no fluids due to treatment.

Until you are in the situation, you probably thought this was not a reality you could have ever imagined—not being able to have sex. Well, you are now living with this new reality. You are still a man, still a part of society, but you may have temporary or permanent loss of sexual function. A new day came with the introduction of Viagra, the little blue pill that makes erections a reality with or without having any sexual hormones in your body. However, without your own sexual hormones, the physical act is not as fulfilling as it probably once was.

Viagra, the blue wonder, is powerful and geared to assist men with erectile dysfunction; it's helpful for men with all types of erectile dysfunction. The way it works is that is helps the blood vessels in the penis relax and thus increases the flow of blood to the area. It has been studied thoroughly, including on more than 3,700 people in clinical trials. Over five million patients use it today. Viagra should be taken about one hour before a sexual encounter but can work up to four hours. It works best on an empty stomach and has minimal side effects. The disadvantages may include headache, upset stomach, and temporary bluish or blurred vision. Ask your doctor about this drug, as it may be helpful for you and your sex life during your prostate cancer treatment.

LOVE TRANSFORMS

Life is not a finished action.
Love is not a complete thought.

—Teilhard de Chardin

The joy and power of love is one of the profound wonders of human existence. When you have love in your life and in your heart, all other struggles are diminished because there is a sense of fullness in your soul. This fullness is always there to draw on when needed, no matter how difficult the situation. Living a life in love makes all the other aspects of life more complete, more acceptable, and more understandable. Even cancer can be easier to live with when there is love.

Love between a couple is fueled by the intimacy they are able to develop and nurture. Knowing you can tell your partner anything about how you feel and he or she will not judge you but love you gives endless joy to the soul. It allows you to be exactly who you are and not try to make excuses. A person in love accepts the past, appreciates the moment, and anticipates the future.

Love manifests itself in many ways. Jim was always there with a kind word, gentle touch, or a warm embrace. He always seems to know what to do to to comfort me, make me feel safe and secure, and know I am loved. In my way I try to demonstrate my love through thoughts, words, and actions. Whether it was setting appointments, meditating each morning, preparing his herbs and vitamins, making a great dinner, or just being there listening to him, it all mattered. Each act is an act of kindness and love, building on our intimate relationship. The conversations about life, death, what is important, family, friends, and the world at large built our relationship and makes it deeper. With cancer, the concern of going deeper in conversations and exposing your innermost feelings no longer seems as fearful. Even discussion of the past and regrets can be worked through during this time. The transformation of the soul and the mind can be magnificent for both partners. Conversations are the building blocks of love and intimacy. Words express love just like actions. They are a direct outcome of our thoughts, even though many times we don't think about how powerful they really are.

Since the emotional ride of cancer is a roller coaster of the highest order, words and their expression in writing can be such an important part of the healing process, a part of letting go of the hurt and letting love enter in its place. I had written a journal on and off throughout my life, so words in short captions were easy for me to put on paper. For me it was a way to reinforce my love for him and give him the support and encouragement we all need in life. For Jim, this was not as simple but more important, because by writing down how he felt, he was able to express himself in ways he had never done before. He was able to get the sense of how truly sensitive he was, how he had such loving feelings for others but had always kept them bottled up inside. The release of these feelings through cards and notes let him get closer to others and, at the same time, get closer to himself.

While we are no poets, here are a few samples of notes we have shared with each other during the past three years during our circle of healing. We have written them to each other and have well over one hundred between us. This was a way for us to capture the moment and the emotion and release it all onto paper.

Words of Love

The meeting of two personalities is like the contact of two chemical substances: if there is any reaction, both are transformed.

—C. G. Jung

Julia to Jim

Mirage (Winter first year of disease)

Dreaming of you—
Your gentle touch
Your loving kiss
Your beautiful face
Your warm embrace

Desiring you—
In any way
On any day
Now and all ways

I love you Jim—You are my mirage—so if perception is
reality, what a great mirage you are! J

Jim to Julia

Learning (Summer)

I love you . . .
We're off to Ann Arbor!
I love to travel with you.
We will learn and see so many things we don't know we
don't know
To life and learning

Thank you so much for the new razor
You're fabulous Love Jim (RLJ)

P.S. XOXOXO

Jim to Julia

Birthday (Fall)

I am not sure what to say . . . but let's start with I love you.
We are about to fly to Hawaii to spend the next week
    celebrating your birthday
(and of course my radiation and 0.03 PSA).

I want you to know how much I love you
You and I are great partners and best friends. I am so
    excited about next week!
Happy Birthday and Congratulations!!
You are the love of my life.

Why I love you
You're my very best friend
You're my soul mate
You're an incredible human being
You're beautiful
You' re so thoughtful and loving
You love me too . . .

How much I love you
You are the love of my life
As big as the Pacific Ocean
As much as each grain of sand on Lanai
As big as the whole universe
38 times more this week than last week

Happy Birthday Week!! Love Jim

Jim to Julia

Baseball (Spring one year later)

Spring is for picnics
And the "boys of summer."
We must do both . . .

Thanks for being my friend.
You are an amazing woman.
I love you . . .

Julia to Jim

Appreciation (Summer)

With each day that passes, I thank God for our love.
Thank you for loving me.

What amazes me about the last few weeks is how close I
    feel to you.
Even though you have so much going on inside and
could easily seem so far away.

Our conversations, our love, our friendship, and
our partnership means so much to me.

You make me laugh, make me cry, make me happy and
always bring me joy.
You have made me feel life, feel love. It is magical.

As our journey continues,
with each moment that passes,
my prayer is we continue to learn more,
be better each day and bring joy into the universe.

Time passes
tomorrow will come before we know it.
I am so proud of you keeping balance in your life
and our life.

I want you to love me now and forever.
To our love
Always J

Julia to Jim

A Valentine Heart (Winter two years later)

Somehow it is so appropriate to focus on hearts
on Valentines Day!
They are symbolic of the pulse of life,
the strength of love and the unending beat of passion.

You have my heart, treasure it, nurture it, and
keep it going strong.
I love loving you with my whole being.
This is the best experience of my life . . .

Kisses and hugs
my love
Julia

"my heart knows no words only feelings—
in any language —I love you
expressed through my thoughts, my actions and deepest
    emotions—
you are priceless, thank you for loving me—
and letting my heart experience such joy—
Jim, you are the joy in my life"

Julia to Jim

Rising (Spring)

Happy Easter!
This is time for a new rising and a rebirth
God knows I am ready for it and all the goodness and
glory that comes with the New Dawn!

Thank you for reminding me the glass is half full—
Like usual I just want it to be totally full!
Why should that surprise you!

I love you—You are my very best friend and life mate.
XOX Julia

Jim to Julia

Happy Day (Fall)

The word growth means "gaining new experience."
Thank you for a wonderful trip to Hong Kong and Tokyo.
It meant so much to be
There with you.
The world is full of so much to learn about and share.

You mean so very much to me.
Love Jim

Julia to Jim

Emotions (Winter three years later)

It is President's Day and the sun is shining.
I have been transformed, you have been transformed, and
we have been transformed—for the better.
You have helped me in so many ways.

My heart aches right now and while I have tears in my eyes,
I am happy.
It is such an unusual feeling,
peace, love, joy, and sadness all combined.

To hear your voice, your laugh, to feel you.
Words cannot express how grateful I am to God
for what we have been through in the last few years.
I loved you then,
I love you now,
I will always love you,
Eternally—Julia

The healing goes on daily, and actions such as finding the perfect card, taking time to reflect on how grateful we are to be here,

and showing the love we have in life are a potent elixir for a healing body. No, we are not poets, but for us the words were beautiful and timely. They helped us cope with the pain and the fears we had. It helped us to share our most intimate feelings in a way that added to our conversations and gave us more strength to deal with the struggle.

DEALING WITH INSURANCE

There is the risk you cannot afford to take, and there is the risk you cannot afford not to take.

—Peter Drucker

Jim did not have to worry about health insurance, which allowed him to focus on healing and curing. While it isn't pleasant, insurance is one of the realities of living with a life-threatening disease. It can get very expensive, especially, as in Jim's case, when you are involved in prolonged treatment. Prepare yourself and know you can get through it; even though there may be some financial challenges, the outcome of a healed person is worth all the money in the world.

There are other important insurance considerations if you are involved with a clinical trial. Some clinical trials offer partial care free of charge. For example, the attendance and participation by doctors in Jim's support group was totally free. In other cases, some insurers will not cover certain costs for a new treatment that is under study. Be sure to ask your doctors about any knowledge they may have concerning this before you start treatment. Additionally, how the paperwork gets filed in critical. "Approved" procedures and drugs can help your chances of getting the treatment covered. Lastly, many insurance policies have a specific exclusion for experimental treatment, so try to get as much covered under traditional/approved practice.

We opted to do whatever we could to heal Jim and paid for many of the treatments from our savings. We viewed this as a conscious choice that we made, just like deciding how to spend our other income. We decided Jim's health came first, no matter what the cost. For the first two years of treatment, Jim exceeded the patient level of personal expenses, and insurance started to pay for the hospital portion of his bills in full. However, they did not pay for his additional acupuncture treatments, vitamins, herbs, and other noncovered expenses.

Depending on your economic situation, there are community and hospital assistance programs available. You can get this type of information from your hospitals administrative or accounting departments. Another way to supplement your insurance is to take all the federal income-tax deductions for health care allowed. Things you might overlook include gas mileage for trips for the treatments and doctors' visits, out-of-pocket costs for prescriptions, and meals and travel expenses.

We learned a few other important tips regarding insurance. First, get a copy of your company insurance and disability policies and find out exactly what your coverage includes. Keep careful records. On more than one occasion, we found the insurance company neglected to pay us or the hospital overcharged us. If you err, err on the side of filing and then learn whether it is covered. Don't let the paperwork scare you off. Either do it yourself or find a cancer resource center or social worker to help you. (Often the company you work for or local community organizations can help as well.) Lastly, if your claim is turned down, don't be afraid to file again and, if necessary, get a letter from your doctor justifying the treatment. Be prepared to do a lot of paper work and get it completed as thoroughly as possible.

SAMPLE LETTER TO APPLY FOR DISABILITY

To Whom It may Concern:

Enclosed are the insurance forms you requested to be completed concerning my patient, _________________________________ (social security no. ___________________). Additionally, I have attached relevant lab reports and tests.

Based upon the nature of Mr. _______________ condition, he will be continuing medical treatment with chemo/hormone therapy. I am recommending long-term disability for Mr. __________ as long as he is engaged in the chemo/hormone therapy and under our care here at _______________________________.

Mr. _______________has advanced-stage high-risk aggressive (describe the condition here) prostate cancer that is probably metastatic, and his current condition warrants this recommendation.

Please contact my office if you require additional documentation. My telephone number and address are the following:

Thank you for your attention to this matter.

Sincerely,

_____________________, M.D.

SAMPLE MEDICAL DISABILITY FORM

Substantiation of Initial Medical Disability

History

(a) Height _____________ Weight _________

(b) Date symptoms first appeared or accident happened
Mo. _____ Day_____ Yr. _____

(c) Date patient ceased work because of disability
Mo. _____ Day _____ Yr. _____

(d) Has patient ever had same or similar condition? No.____ Yes. _____
State when and describe.

(e) Is condition due to injury or sickness arising out of patient's
employment?
No____Yes _____ Unknown _______

(f) Names and addresses of other treating physicians.

Name _______________________ Address _______________________

Name _______________________ Address _______________________

Diagnosis
(a) Date of last examination   Mo. _____ Day _____Yr. _______

(b) ICD diagnostic code (mandatory) _________________

(c) Diagnosis (including any complications) _________________

(d) Subjective symptoms_________________________________

____

(e) Objective findings (including current X-rays, EKGs, laboratory
data and any clinical findings):_________________

(f) Other disease or infirmity affecting present condition_________

____

Dates of Treatment
(a) Date of first visit   Mo. _____ Day _______ Yr. _____

(b) Date of last visit   Mo. ____ Day _______ Yr. _____

(c) Frequency _____Weekly ___Monthly ___Other (specify) _____

____

(d) Is patient still under your care for this condition?
_____Yes _____No, indicate date service terminated. ______________

Nature of Treatment
Include type and date of surgery and medications prescribed, if any.

Progress
(a) Patients has ____Recovered ____Improved ____Stabilized
____Retrogressed

(b) Patient is ____Ambulatory ____House confined ___Bed confined
___Hospital confined

(c) Has patient been hospital confined?
___No ___Yes. Give name and address of hospital ______________

Confined from __________________ through __________________

Limitations
(a) What are patient's present capabilities? ______________

(b) What are present limitations (physical and/or mental)? _____

(c) What restrictions are placed on patient? ______________

Physical Impairment
___ Class 1 No limitations of functional capacity; capable of heavy work. No restrictions.

___ Class 2 Medium manual activity.

___ Class 3 Slight limitations of functional capacity; capable of light work.

___ Class 4 Moderate limitation of functional capacity; capable of clerical/administrative (sedentary) activity.

___ Class 5 Severe limitation of functional capacity; incapable of minimal (sedentary) activity.

Remarks: ____

Mental/Nervous Impairment (If applicable)
(a) Please define "stress" as it applies to this claimant.

(b) What stress and problems in interpersonal relations has claimant had on job?

Remarks:

Do you believe the patient is competent to endorse checks and direct the use of proceeds thereof? _____ No ______Yes

Prognosis
(a) What is the patient's prognosis?

(b) When do you feel patient's maximum medical improvement will be reached?

__1 mo. __1–3 mos. __3–6 mos. __6–9 mos. __1 yr. or longer______

(c) What is the estimated date of the patient's return to work (if any)?_____________________

(d) Do you consider the patient to be a viable candidate for job retraining (Rehabilitation Services)?

_____Yes ___No, please explain________________

____

Remarks

Your hospital and doctors can be your allies in dealing with insurance companies because they want to be paid promptly. Financial help available or monthly payment plans may be available: contact one of the following: a hospital financial counselor, the hospital social worker, patient representatives at the hospital and hospital patient advocates.

If you do not have insurance, there are financial-assistance plans available at most major hospitals. You can apply and still get treatments even if you do not have financial or insurance resources. Local cancer organizations and community outreach programs can help. Call your local community-service cancer representative's office for assistance.

THE THOUSAND-DAY MILESTONE

The life, which is not examined, is not worth living.

—Plato

Over three years ago we were in London. As we ran through Hyde Park, we were running for our lives. Jim had just learned he had serious prostate cancer. We were overwhelmed with fear and sadness, but committed to still living every day to the fullest. It was Jim's birthday and we were going to celebrate it, no matter what.

Three years later we returned to London and reflected on the differences between the two trips.

TIME AND SPACE REALITY

Global location	London	London
Time	March 1998	April 2001
Place	Intercontinental	Four Seasons
Professional space	Corporate executive	Doctoral candidate
Financial	Just fine	Just fine
Mental	Stress and exhaustion	Happy & healthier everyday
Physical	Strong but vulnerable	Stronger every day
Family	Removed/distant	Committed/sharing
Spirituality	Believe in God	Trust in God
Prostate cancer	PSA 39.5	PSA < 0.2
Prognosis	Life threatening	Healed & cured

How long has it been? Over one thousand days, but look at what happened to us. We would love you to learn from our experience. Our goal is to help you become cured and healed from prostate cancer. Commit to yourself, your mind, your soul, and your whole body. Challenge your body and mind once again to work together as one to achieve healing. Be united and unafraid, train yourself to reach for the greatest results, and, as a result, challenge death and accomplish the miracle of living in spite of life's challenges. Strive for a resurrection, for a meaning to and a purpose in life. It is through the unity of the mind, body, and spirit—the three working together—that healing begins at its very essence. Acknowledge that you desire to heal and then continue on the journey—the marathon journey of healing.

Some talk about a marathon race being 26.2 miles long, but those involved in the marathon of treating and healing cancer do go the distance. The marathon starts and you don't really understand what's happening, and then it becomes all that matters. That first day, month, year, two years amount to tens of thousands of hours. This is a true marathon, a marathon for life–definitely the most meaningful one of our lives. To Jim, the marathon has been worth every single step, every moment, every day. Prepare to exert yourself, and look for joy in the unexpected outcomes of the journey.

The world is an uncertain place, but what counts is your life, your family and friends, and your willingness to commit every day to being the best in life. When time and space seems dull or devoid of meaning, we have been given the chance to grab hold of life, reverse a downward spiral, and move on to a new, thrilling circle of life. Jim and I are grateful—we took it all in, we moved on. The struggle is worth every moment, the struggle is what life is and why we are here to live and learn in times of both sickness and wellness.

CLOSING THOUGHTS

Often people attempt to live their lives backwards: they try to have more things, or more money, in order to do more of what they want to so that they will be happier. The way it actually works is the reverse. You must first be who you really are, then, do what you need to do, in order to have what you want.

—Margaret Young

Cancer is a terrible disease. Cancer can kill you. Cancer will change your life. Prostate cancer forces you to make dramatic choices in your life. You can make it through the journey no matter how challenging it may be.

You learn more about living when you are confronted with dying and your own mortality. While this is not an experience you want anyone to go through, there are significant lessons that come with cancer. You will learn more about yourself, your family and friends, your work, and your life because of the disease. It forces you to ask the really difficult questions in life we normally are too busy to ask. Questions like, What is really important to me? What do I want to do with the rest of my life? What is more important to me, the quality or the quantity of my life—or a combination of both? By answering these questions for yourself your world will seem much more fulfilled and complete, because you are consciously making choices about how you are living your life rather than just going through the motions.

While it may be difficult, you will learn more about life by facing the reality of potential death. The Circle of Healing is ongoing and Jim and I have been transformed by it. It is an experience that we will never forget. What we have taken away from all of this is appreciation.

Appreciation of the abundance life has brought to us.
Appreciation of our doctors, healers and supporters
Appreciation of our family and friends
Appreciation of our health
Appreciation of ourselves
Appreciation of our personal and spiritual growth

Appreciation of hope
Appreciation of our love
Appreciation of life
Appreciation of each moment

What became most important to us is to live a life in love, to give and receive love freely to and from ourselves and the world around us. The rest of life is the background noise that only makes it all seem worthwhile. In closing, this is not really an ending of the journey for us. It is actually a new beginning, and we are grateful to be here now in life, and more in love than ever.

For the tears passed
For the fears surpassed
For the journey unknown
We are now home
Body, mind, and soul as one
We learn that with love
All is fine
Now and throughout time

For a long time it had seemed to me that life was about to begin—real life. But there was always some obstacle in the way, something to be got through first, some unfinished business, time still to be served, and a debt to be paid. Then life would begin. At last it dawned on me that these obstacles were my life.

—Alfred D'Souza

APPENDIX

Glossary

Adjuvant chemotherapy—One or more anticancer drugs used in combination with surgery or radiation therapy as part of the treatment of cancer. *Adjuvant* usually means "in addition to" initial treatment.

Adrenal glands—Two glands located above the kidneys (one above each kidney). They produce several kinds of hormones, including a small amount of sex hormones.

Antiandrogen—A drug that blocks the action of male sex hormones.

Antibody—A protein produced by a plasma cell in the lymphatic system or bone marrow. An antibody binds to the specific antigen that has stimulated the immune system. Once bound, other cells of the immune system can destroy the antigen. See *Immune system.*

Antigen—A substance, foreign to the body, that stimulates the production of antibodies by the immune system. Antigens include foreign proteins, bacteria, viruses, pollen, and other materials.

Anus—The opening at the lower end of the rectum through which solid waste leaves the body.

Benign—Not cancerous.

Benign porstatic hyperplasia—A noncancerous condition in which an overgrowth of prostate tissue pushes against the urethra and the bladder, blocking the flow of urine. Also called benign prostatic hypertrophy, or BPH.

Biological therapy—Use of biologicals (substances produced by our own cells) or biological response modifiers (substances that affect the patient's defense systems) in the treatment of cancer.

Biopsy—A surgical procedure that involves taking small samples of tissue in order to test them.

Biopsy blast—A gun used to gather samples from tissue. Somewhat painful, but very informative in diagnosis.

Bladder—The hollow organ that stores urine.

Blood count—Measurement of the number of red cells, white cells, and platelets in a sample of blood.

Bone marrow—The inner, spongy core of bone that produces blood cells.

Cancer—A general term for more than 100 diseases characterized by abnormal and uncontrolled growth of cells. The resulting mass, or tumor, can invade and destroy surrounding normal tissues. Cancer cells from the tumor can spread through the blood or lymph to start new cancers in other parts of the body.

Chemotherapy—Treatment with anticancer drugs.

Clinical trial—The systematic investigation of the effects of materials or methods, according to a formal study plan and generally in a human population with a particular disease or class of diseases. In cancer research, a clinical trial generally refers to the evaluation of treatment methods, such as surgery, drugs, or radiation techniques, although methods of prevention, detection, or diagnosis may be the subject of such studies.

Colon—The last four to five feet of the digestive tract. The colon absorbs water and minerals from digested material.

Combination chemotherapy—Use of two or more anticancer drugs.

Combination therapy—The use of two or more modes of treatment—surgery, radiotherapy, chemotherapy, immunotherapy—in combination, alternately or together, to achieve optimum results against cancer.

Control group—In clinical studies, this is a group of patients that receives *standard treatment,* a treatment or intervention currently being used and considered to be of proved effectiveness on the basis of past studies. Results in patients receiving newly developed treatments may then be compared to the control group. In cases where no standard treatment yet exists for a particular condition, the control group would receive no treatment. No patient is placed in a control group without treatment if there is any beneficial treatment known for that patient.

Cryosurgery—A procedure that uses extremely cold liquid nitrogen to destroy cancer cells.

Cystoscopy—A procedure in which the doctor inserts a lighted instrument through the urethra (the tube leading from the bladder to the outside of the body) to look inside the bladder.

Digital rectal exam (DRE)—Insertion of a doctor's protected and gloved finger into the rectum. Often done to determine how the tumor feels and if it is large enough to feel.

Double-blind—Characteristic of a controlled experiment in which neither the patient nor the attending physician knows whether the patient is getting one or another drug or dose. In *single-blind* studies, patients do not know which of several treatments they are receiving, thus preventing personal bias from influencing their reactions and study results. In either case, the treatment can be quickly identified, if necessary, by a special code.

Dry orgasm—Sexual climax without the release of semen.

Ejaculation—The release of semen through the penis during orgasm.

Estrogen—A female sex hormone.

External radiation—Use of a machine to aim high-energy rays at the cancer.

Genitourinary system—The parts of the body that play a role in reproduction, getting rid of waste products in the form of urine, or both.

Grade—How closely a tumor resembles normal tissue of its same type. Suggests the tumor's most likely rate of growth. In prostate cancer, this may be referred to as the Gleason grade.

Grade (Gleason grade)—Predicts a tumor's aggressiveness (seriousness) based on its appearance under a microscope. Based on a grading system, defined by Gleason, ranging from 1 to 10.

Hormone—Chemical product of the endocrine glands of the body, which, when secreted into body fluids, has a specific effect on other organs. Hormones control the actions of certain cells or organs.

Hormone therapy—Treatment that prevents cancer cells from getting the hormones they need to grow. Hormone therapy for prostate cancer keeps the cancer cells from getting male hormones. Treatment may involve removing the testicles or giving female hormones or other drugs to prevent the production of male hormones or to block their effect on cancer cells.

Imaging tests—Tests that produce pictures of the inside of the body to help diagnose and stage prostate cancer.

Immune system—A complex network of organs, cells, and specialized substances distributed throughout the body and defending it from foreign invaders that cause infection or disease.

Immunotherapy—A form of biological therapy. An experimental method of treating cancer, using substances, that stimulate the body's immune defense system.

Impotence—Inability to have an erection.

Incision—A cut made during surgery.

Incontinence—Inability to control the flow of urine from the bladder.

Inflammation—A response to tissue injury that causes redness, swelling and pain.

Informed consent—The process in which a patient learns about and understands the purpose and aspects of a clinical trial and then agrees to participate. Of course, a patient may decline to participate. This process includes a document defining how much a patient must know about the potential benefits and risks of therapy before being able to agree to undergo it knowledgeably. (Informed consent is required by federally conducted, funded, or regulated studies as well as by many state laws.) If a patient signs an informed consent form and enters a trial, he or she is still free to leave the trial at any time and can receive other available medical care.

Interferon—A protein substance produced by white blood cells and other types of cells that have been exposed to certain viruses. In test animals, interferon has shown some activity against tumors. Studies of its usefulness in treating some types of human cancer are under way. One of a number of new agents available as biological therapy.

Internal radiation—The placement of radioactive material inside the body as close as possible to the cancer.

Intravenous pyelogram—X-rays of the kidneys, ureters, and bladder taken after a dye is injected into a vein. Also called IVP.

Investigational new drug—A drug approved by the Food and Drug Administration for use in clinical trials but not for commercial marketing.

Investigator—An investigator is the experienced clinical researcher who prepares a protocol or treatment plan and implements it with patients.

Local therapy—Treatment that affects cancer cells only in the treated area.

Luteinizing hormone-releasing hormone (LHRH) agonist—A substance that closely resembles luteinizing hormone-releasing hormone (LHRH), which controls the production of sex hormones. However, LHRH agonists affect the body differently than does LHRH. The agonists keep the testicles from producing hormones.

Lymph nodes—Small, bean-shaped organs located along the channels of the lymphatic system. Bacteria or cancer cells that enter the lymphatic system may be found in the lymph nodes. Also called lymph glands.

Lymphatic system—The tissues and organs, including the bone marrow, spleen, thymus, and lymph nodes, that produce and store cells that fight infection and disease.

Malignant—Cancerous; can spread to other parts of the body.

Metastasis—The transfer of disease from one part of the body to another. In cancer, metastasis is the migration of cancer cells from the original tumor site through the blood and lymph vessels to produce cancers in other tissues. Metastasis is the term used for a secondary cancer growing at a distant site.

Monoclonal antibodies—One of several new substances used in biological therapy. These antibodies, all exactly alike, are mass-produced and designed to home in on target cancer cells. Monoclonal antibodies are products of new scientific techniques and may prove useful in both cancer diagnosis and treatment.

Multimodality therapy—The combined use of more than one method of treatment—for example, surgery and chemotherapy.

Oncologist—A doctor who specializes in treating cancer. Some oncologists specialize in a particular type of cancer treatment. For example, a radiation oncologist treats cancer with radiation.

Orchiectomy—Surgery to remove the testicles.

Palpable tumor—A tumor that can be felt in a digital rectal exam.

Pathologist—A doctor who identifies diseases by studying cells and tissues under a microscope.

Pelvic—Referring to the areas of the body located below the waist and surrounded by the hip and pubic bones.

Placebo—An inactive substance resembling a medication, given for psychological effect or as a control in evaluating a medicine believed to be active. It is usually a tablet, capsule or injection that contains a harmless substance but appears to be the same as the medicine being tested. A placebo may be compared with a new drug when no one knows if any drug or treatment will be effective.

Polyp—A grapelike shaped or mushroomlike growth that occurs on the lining of the colon and rectum. Polyps can change over time, from benign to cancer growth. They should be identified and removed.

Polyposis—A condition in which the colon is lined with many polyps.

Prognosis—The probable outcome or course of a disease; the chance of recovery.

Prostate—A male sex gland; it produces fluid that forms part of semen.

Prostatectomy—Surgery to remove part of the prostate. Removal of the entire prostate is called radical prostatectomy, which is performed two ways. Retropubic prostatectomy is the surgical removal of the prostate through an incision in the abdomen. Perineal prostatectomy is surgery to remove the prostate through an incision made between the scrotum and the anus.

Prostate-specific antigen—A protein produced by the prostate gland and found at low levels in the blood. Its level goes up in the blood of some men who have prostate cancer, benign prostatic hyperplasia, or prostatitis. called PSA.

PSA (prostate-specific antigen) blood test—A key measure used by doctors to measure the level of prostate-specific antigens in the blood.

The higher it is, the potentially larger the problem. Anything over 20 is very serious. Ideally PSA is under 2.

PSAD (PSA density)—A measure of the concentration of PSA in the blood.

Prostatic acid phosphatase—An enzyme produced by the prostate. Its level in the blood goes up in some men who have prostate cancer. Called PAP.

Protocol—The outline or plan for use of an experimental procedure or experimental treatment.

Radiation therapy—Treatment using high-energy X-rays, cobalt-60, radium, neutrons, or other types of cell-destroying radiation (called radiotherapy) used to kill cancer cells.

Radiosensitizers—Drugs being studied to try to boost the effect of radiation therapy.

Randomized clinical trials—A study in which patients with similar traits, such as extent of disease, are chosen or selected by chance to be placed in separate groups that are comparing different treatments. Because irrelevant factors or preferences do not influence the distribution of patients, the treatment groups can be considered comparable and results of the different treatments used in different groups can be compared. (There is no way at the time for the researchers to know which of the treatments is best. It is the patient's choice to be in a randomized trial or not.) (See also *Clinical trials.*)

Rectal exam—a procedure, in which a doctor inserts a gloved, lubricated finger into the rectum and feels the prostate through the wall of the rectum to check the prostate for hard or lumpy areas.

Rectum—The last six to eight inches of the large intestine and the lowest part of the colon. The rectum stores solid waste until it leaves the body through the anus.

Recur—To return after cancer treatment has been completed.

Regression—The state of growing smaller or disappearing; used to describe the shrinkage or disappearance of a cancer.

Remission—Disappearance of the signs and symptoms of cancer. When this happens, the disease is said to be "in remission." Remission can be temporary or permanent.

Risk—the possibility of a person developing a certain disease.

Risk benefit Ratio—The relation between the risks and benefits of a given treatment or procedure. Institutional Review Boards (IRBs), located where the clinical trial is to take place, determine that the risks in a study are reasonable with respect to the potential benefits.

It is up to the patient to decide if it is reasonable for him or her to take part in a study.

RT-PCR test—reverse transcriptase-poly chain-reaction test.

Screening—Identifies people without symptoms who may have a disease.

Scrotum—The external pouch of skin that contains the testicles.

Semen—The fluid that is released through the penis during orgasm. Semen is made up of sperm from the testicles and fluid from the prostate and other sex glands.

Side effect—A secondary and usually adverse effect, as from a drug or other treatment. For example, nausea is a side effect of some anti-cancer drugs.

Stage—Describes the extent of the prostate cancer's spread in the prostate and throughout the body. For those more official types, it is referred to as the TNM Staging System.

Staging—Doing exams or tests to learn the extent of a cancer, especially whether it has spread from its original site to other parts of the body.

Standard treatment—A treatment or other intervention currently being used and considered to be of proved effectiveness on the basis of past studies.

Study arm—Patients in clinical trials are assigned to one part or segment of a study—a study "arm." One arm receives a different treatment from another.

Surgery—An operation.

Systemic therapy—Treatment that reaches and affects cancer cells all over the body.

Testicles—The two egg-shaped glands that produce sperm and male hormones.

Testosterone—A male sex hormone.

Therapeutic—Pertaining to treatment.

Transurethral resection of the prostate—The use of an instrument inserted through the penis to remove tissue from the prostate. Also called TURP or TUR.

TRUS (transrectal ultrasound)—An imaging technique that uses sound waves and their echoes to map the prostate.

Tumor—An abnormal mass of tissue. Can be benign or malignant.

Ultrasonography—A test in which sound waves (called ultrasound) are bounced off tissues, and the echoes are converted into a picture (sonogram).

Urethra—The tube that carries urine or semen to the outside of the body.

Urologist—A doctor who specializes in diseases of the urinary organs in females and the urinary and sex organs in males.

Vasectomy—Surgery performed to sterilize a man by cutting the vas deferens, a tube that transports sperm.

Charts and Forms

SAMPLE MEDICAL RECORD

MY NAME

HEIGHT   WEIGHT   DATE OF BIRTH   AGE AT DIAGNOSIS

PRIMARY PHYSICIAN   PHONE

UROLOGIST   PHONE

ONCOLOGIST   PHONE

PRINTED REPORTS TO INCLUDE IN YOUR FILE

- MEDICAL HISTORY / PHYSICIAL EXAMINATION FINDINGS
- OPERATIVE PROCEDURE REPORTS (IF APPLICABLE)
- DNA FLOW CYTOMETRY RESULTS
- PROPOSED TREAMENT PLANS

DIGAGNOSTIC STUDIES

- PSA BLOOD TESTS
- TRANSRECTAL ULTRASOUND EXAMS
- CHEST X-RAYS
- BONE SCAN & BONE X-RAYS
- CT/MRI SCANS—OTHER

IMPORTANT INFORMATION FOR INITIAL TREATMENT DECISION

INITIAL PSA VALUE _____ (normal range _____)

DETECTION   PALPABLE NODULE BY DIGITAL RECTAL EXAM?
      YES   NO

URINARY OBSTRUCTION SYMPTOME PRESENT?
      YES   NO

FROM BIOPSY, GLEASON GRADE: (____ + ____ = ________ SCORE)

DIAGNOSIS

DNA PLOIDY ANALYSIS: DIPLOID
ANEUPLOID   TETRAPLOID

TUMOR VOLUME ______ cubic centimeters

WAS PSA MORE THAN 4 TIMES THE UPPER
LIMIT OF NORMAL?   YES   NO

DO TRUS, CT, and/or MRI SCANS SUGGEST TUMOR
IS STILL CONFINED TO GLAND?   YES   NO
WAS PELVIC LYMPH NODE DISSECTION NEGA-
TIVE FOR METASTATIC INVOLVEMENT?
YES   NO

IS BONE SCAN NEGATIVE FOR ANY EVIDENCE
OF METASTATIS?   YES   NO

EVALUATION

IF BONE SCAN IS ABNORMAL, DO X-RAYS
RULE OUT TUMOR(S)?   YES   NO

A1: Unsuspected, not palpable;   STAGE A
involves <5% of specimen;
Gleason <5

A1: Unsuspected, not palpable;
involves <5% of specimen;
Gleason = or >5

B1: Palpable tumor, involves only   STAGE B
One lobe of gland, tumor <2cm in
diameter

B2: Palpable tumor(s). One tumor 2 cm
or larger, or tumor in both lobes

Tumor invades through gland   STAGE C
capsule; "positive" margin at
resection, and/or seminal vesicle
involvement

D1: Spread to nearby lymph nodes   STAGE D

D2: Spread to distant lymph nodes,
bones, lungs, and/or other organs

Valuable Resources

Best Doctors
Worldwide Healthcare Services
1359 Silver Bluff Road, Suite F-2
Aiken, SC 29803
Telephone: 800-675-1199
Fax: 803-648-7240
E-mail: *info@bestdoctors.com*
Web site: *www.bestdoctors.com*

CapCure
1250 Fourth Street, Suite 360
Santa Monica, CA 90401
Telephone: 310-458-2873, 800-757-2873
Fax: 310-418-8079
E-mail: *capcure@capcure.org*
Web site: *www.capcure.org*
National Cancer Institute (NCI)
Cancer Information Service: 800-422-6237
Web site: *www.nci.nih.gov*

PAACT (Patient Advocates for Advanced Cancer Treatments)
1143 Parmelee N.W., Grand Rapids, MI 49504
P.O. Box 141695
Grand Rapids, MI 49514
Telephone: 616-453-1477
Fax: 616-453-1846
Web site: *www.paactusa.org*
E-mail: *paact@paactusa.org*

Prostate Forum
P.O. Box 6696
Charlottesville, VA 22906
Telephone: 804-974-1313
Fax: 804-974-9597
E-mail: *myers@esinet.net*

Web site: *www.prostateforum.com*
Subscription rates: Individual, $46/yr.; Institution, $75/yr.
Health Insurance Association of America (HIAA)
1025 Connecticut Avenue, N.W., Suite 1200
Washington, DC 10036—3998
Web site: *www.hiaa.org*

CANCER National Insurance Consumer: 800-942-4242.

General Information Web sites
Achoo, Internet Health Care Directory—*www.achoo.com*
CancerNet—Maintained by National Cancer Institute—*http://cncernet.nci.nih.gov*
Commonweal—*www.commonwealhealth.org*
Doctor's Guide to Prostate Cancer—*www.pslgroup.com/prostcancer.htm;* An excellent source of prostate cancer news and information.
Enter the Circle—*http://rattler.cameron.edu/circle*
Food and Drug Administration—*www.fda.gov*
Healthfinder—U.S. Dept. of Health and Human Services; information on on-line publications, clearinghouses, databases, Web-sites, and support and self-help groups. *www.healthfinder.gov.*
Healthgate—Source of health, wellness and biomedical information. *www.healthgate.com*
International Cancer Alliance—*www.icare.org*
International Impotence Education Month—*www.iiem.org*
James Buchanan Brady Urological Institute, Johns Hopkins Hospital—*http://prostate.urol.jhu.edu*
Medicine On-Line—Patient and professional educational information. *www.meds.com*
Medinfo.org Oncology Resources—*www.medinfo.org*
Memorial Sloan-Kettering Cancer Center—*www.mskcc.org*
Physician's Guide to the Internet—*www.webcom.com/pgi/*
Prostate Cancer—*www.prostatecancer.com*
Prostate Cancer Discussion—Send e-mail to *listserv@sjuvm.stjohns.edu;* message: subscription: leave name and e-mail address.
Prostate Health Registry and Patient Information Source—An official Web site of the Prostate Health Council of the AFUD *www.prostatehealth.com/*

Prostate Pointers—Award-winning prostate cancer information site, maintained by prostate-cancer survivors. *www.prostatepointers.org/prostate*

Reuters Health Information Service—Daily press releases; *www.reutershealth.com*

University of Michigan Prostate Cancer Home Page—*www.cancer. med.umich.edu/prostean/prostean.html*

Virgil's Prostate Online—*www.prostate-online.com*

Clinical Trials

Centerwatch—*www.centerwatch.com*

MD Anderson Clinical Trials—*www.clinicaltrials.org*

National Cancer Institute Clinical Trials—*http://cancernet.nci.nih.gov trials/h_clinic.htm*

Patient Clinical Trials: PDQ (Physician Data Query, a service of the National Cancer Institute)—*http://cancernet.nci.nih.gov/prot/protsrch. html*; includes international trials.

Publications

Cancer Online—Full-text electronic implementation of CANCER, an Interdisciplinary International Journal of the American Cancer Society; *www.interscience.wiley.com/jpages/0008—543X.*

Journal of the American Medical Association (JAMA)—*www.jama.com*

Journal of Urology—*www.jurology.com*

New England Journal of Medicine— *http://content.nejm.org*

The Urology Channel—Electronic journal for physicians. Lay visitors are admitted on an honor system, but are expected to register. This group does not respond to request for medical advice or referrals. *www.chronicle.org/uro.htm*

Organizations

American Cancer Society—*www.cancer.org*

American Foundation for Urologic Disease—*www.afud.org*

American Institute for Cancer Research—*www.aicr.org*

American Medical Association—*www.ama-assn.org*

American Prostate Society—*www.ameripros.org*

American Urologic Association—*www.auanet.org*

Cancerlit—E-mail: *listserv@wvm.edu*

CapCURE—*www.capcure.org*

Education Center for Prostate Cancer Patients (ECPCP)—*www.ecpcp.org*

Mediconsult—*www.mediconsult.com/prostate*
Man to Man—*www.cancer.org/m2m/m2m.html*
Mathews Foundation for Prostate Cancer Research—*www.mathews.org*
Men's Health Network—*www.menshealthnetwork.org*
National Cancer Institute—*www.nci.nih.gov*
National Coalition for Cancer Survivorship—*www.cansearch.org*
National Prostate Cancer Coalition (NPCC)—*www.4npcc.org*
Patient Advocates for Advanced Cancer Treatment (PAACT)—*www.paactusa.org*
USTOO! International—*www.ustoo.com*

Spanish Resources
National Cancer Institute (NCI) Cancernet Database—*http://imsdd. meb.unibonn.de/cancernet/cancernet.html*
WWW Cancer—*www.arc.com/cancernet/cancernet.html*

REFERENCES

American Foundation for Urological Disease. (1997). *Prostate cancer resource guide.*

American Gastrointerological Association. (1998). *Colorectal screening brochure.* Bethesda, MD: Author.

Anderson, G. (1993). *50 Essential things to do when the doctor says its cancer.* New York: Penguin Books U.S.A.

Balch, J. & Balch, P. (1990). *Prescription for nutritional healing.* Garden City, NY: Avery Publishing Group.

Bostwick, D., Larson, T. & MacLennan. (1996). *Prostate cancer.* New York: Villard Books.

Chopra, D. (1994). *Journey into healing.* New York: Crown Publishers, Inc.

Clapp, L. (1997). *Prostate health in 90 days.* Carlsbad, CA: Hay House, Inc.

Colter, A. (1999). *From this moment on.* New York: Random House.

Connelly, D. (1994). *Traditional acupuncture.* Columbia, MD: Traditional Acupuncture Institute.

Creighton, J., Matthews-Simonton, S. & Simonton, O. (1978). *Getting well again.* New York: Bantam.

Elias, J. & Ketcham, K. (1998). *The five elements of self-healing.* New York: Harmony Books.

Epstein, D. (1994). *The 12 stages of healing.* San Rafael, CA, and Novato, CA: Amber Allen Publishing and New World Library.

Ford, D. (1998). *The dark side of the light chasers.* New York: Riverhead Books.

Gardinier, E. (1997). *How I conquered cancer.* Houston, TX: Emerald Ink Publishers.

Gersh, W., Golden, W. & Robbins, D. (1997). *Mind over malignancy.* Oakland, CA: New Harbinger Publications.

Hadady, Letha. (1996). *Asian health secrets.* New York: Three Rivers Press.

Hay, L. (1994). *You can heal your life.* Carlsbad, CA: Hay House Inc.

Hay, L. (1998). *Heal your body.* Carlsbad, CA: Hay House Inc.

Health Insurance Association of America. *Consumer's guide to disability and insurance.* (Publication no. C104).

Health Insurance Association of America. *Consumer's guide to health insurance.* (Publication no. 003).

Hoffman, B. (1996). *A cancer survivor's almanac.* Minneapolis, MN: Chronimed Publishing.

Institute for Personality and Ability Testing. (1978). *Images of cancer: a diagnostic tool for the process of disease.* Champaign, IL: Author.

King, J. & Pearlroth, J. (1998). *Cancer combat.* New York: Bantam Books.

Lewis, J. & Berger, R. (1997). *New guidelines for surviving prostate cancer.* Westbury, NY: Health Education Literary Publisher.

Moyad, M. & Oesterling, J. (1997). *The ABCs of prostate cancer.* Lanham, MD: Madison Books.

Moyers, B. (1993). *Healing and the mind.* New York: Doubleday.

National Institutes of Health. (1996). *What you need to know about prostate cancer.* (Publication no. 96—1576).

National Institutes of Health. (1997). *Facing forward: a guide for cancer survivors.* Washington, DC

National Institutes of Health. (1997). *What are clinical trials all about?* Washington, DC

Ornish, Dean. (1998). *Love and survival.* New York: Harper Collins.

Overholser, L. & Pelton, R. (1994). *Alternatives in cancer therapy.* New York: Fireside.

Reid, D. (1986). *Chinese herbal medicine.* Boston: Shambhala Publications, Inc.

Reid, D. (1995). *The complete book of Chinese health and healing.* Boston: Shambhala Publications, Inc.

Reid, D. (1995). *A handbook of Chinese healing herbs.* Boston: Shambhala Publications, Inc.

Scientific American, Inc. (1997). *What you need to know about cancer.* New York: W.H. Freeman.

Siegel, B. (1986). *Love, medicine & miracles.* New York: Harper & Row.

Stoddard, A. (1986). *Living a beautiful life.* New York: Hearst Corporation.

Stratton, E. (1997). *Seeds of light.* New York: Simon & Schuster.

Taylor, N. (1998). *Green tea.* New York: Kensington Publishing Corp.

Weil, (1995). *Spontaneous healing.* New York: Alfred A. Knopf.

Westen, R. (1998). *10 days to detox.* New York: Doubleday.

Worsley, J. R. (1991). *Talking about acupuncture in New York.* Worcester, England: Billings & Sons.